What You Didn't Think to Ask Your Obstetrician

RAYMOND I. POLIAKIN, M.D.

THIRD EDITION

New York Chicago San Francisco Lisbon London Madrid Mexico City
Milan New Delhi San Juan Seoul Singapore Sydney Toronto

To my lovely wife, Vickie,
who has always given me love and support,
and to Lauren, Natasha, Tess, and Beau,
my four beautiful children

1 2 3 4 5 6 7 8 9 10 11 12 13 14 15 16 17 18 19   FGR/FGR   0 9 8 7 6

ISBN-13: 978-0-07-147226-5
ISBN-10:   0-07-147226-6

McGraw-Hill books are available at special quantity discounts to use as premiums and sales promotions, or for use in corporate training programs. For more information, please write to the Director of Special Sales, Professional Publishing, McGraw-Hill, Two Penn Plaza, New York, NY 10121-2298. Or contact your local bookstore.

This book is printed on acid-free paper.

Contents

About the Author

Raymond Poliakin, M.D., was born and raised in New York City. He received his medical degree from New York Medical College with Alpha Omega Alpha honors and his bachelor's degree in biology from SUNY at Stony Brook. He completed his internship and residency in obstetrics and gynecology at the University of Southern California Medical Center, where he is also a clinical professor emeritus. Dr. Poliakin has been in private practice for over twenty years in Thousand Oaks, California, and has written for *Parents* magazine and *Shape*. He lives with his wife, four teenagers, two dogs, and three cats and enjoys road bicycling and playing guitar.

CHAPTER I

Office Visits and Early Considerations

Q. *How can parents become more involved in the birth process?*

A. I believe that parents should become involved preconception, meaning that their interests in having a healthy pregnancy, a normal labor and delivery, and a healthy baby should begin before the woman becomes pregnant. This preparation should cover many aspects—medical, genetic, physiological, nutritional, and psychological—in conjunction with the health care provider.

Prepare yourself medically. If you have a chronic disease, such as hypertension or a thyroid problem, get it stabilized before attempting a pregnancy. If you are on one or more medications, ask your doctor if it is safe to take them during your pregnancy. You may have to discontinue a certain medicine and change to one that has been shown to be safe to take during pregnancy. Get your annual checkup, Pap smear, and any lab work, tests, or mammogram that are due. Get a dental checkup and any dental work and x-rays before your pregnancy.

Prepare yourself genetically. Be aware of hereditary disorders that are part of your family history, such as muscular dystrophy, or genetic disorders that are part of your ethnic background. Get tested to see if you are a carrier of these disorders as well as for cystic fibrosis. If you test positive as a carrier, have your significant other tested to see if he is a carrier as well. If you are both carriers, consult a genetic counselor.

Prepare yourself physiologically. Begin a new exercise regimen before you become pregnant so you can continue to exercise during your pregnancy. The time to start an exercise program is not after your first prenatal visit. Preconception is also the time for both parents to stop smoking and drinking. The same holds true for your nutritional, or dietary, habits. Begin to eat properly before you become pregnant; lose those extra pounds before you become pregnant. You should also start a prenatal vitamin that contains at least 400 micrograms of folic acid three months prior to becoming pregnant to decrease the risk of neural tube defects in your newborn.

Finally, you and your partner need to become psychologically ready for the pregnancy and your baby. The responsibility of parenting begins with your idea that you both want to have a baby.

Q. *Shouldn't we just trust the physician?*

A. I hope that all patients have trust in their physicians. Certainly, I hope that all my patients trust me. Trust is the cement that bonds patient and doctor. Trust in the physician gives the patient confidence that she will be treated properly and safely throughout her pregnancy and that if a complication does arise, it will be discovered promptly and treated appropriately.

However, blind trust is not a wise approach. No one is perfect, and there may be more than one course of action to take in your treatment. If you are offered only one treatment plan, ask your doctor about alternatives to his or her strategy.

Q. *Is there such a thing as a stupid question?*

A. There is no such thing as a stupid question. A patient is not expected to know everything about her pregnancy and should feel comfortable asking her physician about anything, from the size and weight of her fetus at a certain gestational age to a particularly bothersome symptom or a referral for childbirth classes or a pediatrician.

Q. *How do I choose my doctor?*

A. The first step is to check your insurance plan against the list of obstetricians (OBs) in the area, which you can get from the hospital. Your insurance plan may narrow down your choice of doctors. Next, ask your relatives, friends, hairdressers, or business associates for recommendations. Make sure that they like their doctor.

If you do not have these resources, call the hospital where you plan to deliver. Specifically, call the labor and delivery (L&D) and emergency room (ER) departments for recommendations. Call for recommendations during both the day shift and the night shift. Most hospitals have a policy to recommend three doctors at a time. You will have twelve recommendations, but usually one doctor is named more often than the others. Visit that doctor first.

Q. *Should I set up an appointment to meet the doctor?*

A. If you still aren't sure about your choice of a doctor, set up a consultation with the rest of the physicians on your list. Come prepared with questions. Discuss your pertinent history and any concerns you may have about your pregnancy and labor and delivery. Ask about the doctor's call schedule. What are the chances that this doctor will be the one delivering your baby? If it is a group practice, how often will you be seeing the other doctors? Whose choice is it? Ask about elective inductions and elective cesarean sections (C-sections). Don't ask about C-section rates; there are too many variables. Does the doctor perform ultrasounds, or are you sent out? Are VBACs (vaginal births after cesarean) done? Ask about the use of labor epidurals. Talk to the office manager about insurance and any financial questions. Finally, did you feel comfortable with the doctor?

PRENATAL VISIT

Q. *What happens at the first prenatal visit?*

A. Your doctor will discuss any problems associated with your medical history and basic problems that may arise during your pregnancy. Bring a list of questions that you want answered. Your doctor will prescribe a prenatal vitamin and an omega-3 fatty acid supplement and explain what will happen during your follow-up visits. You will be given an appointment schedule based on your last menstrual period (LMP).

Your weight and blood pressure will be taken and recorded as a baseline. You may be asked to urinate before your pelvic exam because the bladder sits on top of the uterus, and a full bladder makes for both an uncomfortable exam for you and a difficult and sometimes misleading exam for the doctor. A physical exam will be performed, including a breast and pelvic exam. A Pap smear, if due, will be performed. Blood will be taken for the following tests: complete blood count (CBC), VDRL, rubella, blood type, Rh titer, hepatitis B, HIV, and cystic fibrosis carrier status. (More on these tests further down and in Chapter 7.) Routine cultures of your cervix will be taken for gonorrhea and chlamydia, and a vaginal culture and urine culture will be performed.

Q. *Why is the pelvic exam performed?*

A. The pelvic exam tells us many important facts. First, it confirms your pregnancy and the length of your pregnancy thus far. The doctor will also be able to discover any abnormalities of the uterus, such as fibroid tumors (benign tumors of the muscles of the uterus) or congenital abnormalities of the uterus, as well as cysts or tumors of the ovary or the presence of an ectopic pregnancy (see Chapter 8). The doctor will also measure the birth canal and estimate its adequacy for passage of your baby. If any abnormalities are detected or suspected, an ultrasound exam will be performed.

Q. *Do I have pelvic exams during each office visit?*

A. Most physicians perform a pelvic exam during the initial office visit and again at the end of your pregnancy. The pelvic exams at 38 weeks and beyond are used by your doctor to assess the ripeness of your cervix, an indication that your pregnancy is mature and ready for the birth of your baby!

Q. *Why is the urine tested?*

A. The doctor tests the first morning urine for the presence of sugar, protein, and nitrites. About one-sixth of pregnant women will have sugar in their urine normally; however, since this also occurs in diabetes mellitus, a test would then be performed for this disorder. If protein is found in your urine, you may have a problem with your kidneys. The nitrite test screens for a possible urinary tract infection.

Q. *Why is the uterus measured (fundal height)?*

A. The uterus is measured to ascertain proper growth of the fetus and to alert your doctor to any possible problems or unusual circumstances, such as miscarriage, blighted ovum, molar pregnancy, twins, a growth-restricted or overly large fetus, or too little or too much amniotic fluid.

Q. *How is the uterus measured?*

A. Until the 12th week of pregnancy, the uterus is measured by pelvic examination. The uterus can first be felt abdominally at about 14 weeks. Between 14 and 20 weeks, the uterus is measured in relation to the belly button. After 20 weeks, a tape measure is used to measure the distance from the top of your pubic bone to the top of your uterus (the fundus). This length, measured in centimeters, correlates with the week of your pregnancy until the 32nd week.

Q. *When can you first hear the fetal heart tones?*

A. With a medical doptone, an instrument that uses ultrasonic waves, the fetal heart can be heard between 10 and 12 weeks. A store-bought nonprofessional doptone will pick up your baby's heart tones at 18 to 20 weeks.

Q. *How often are the follow-up visits, and what does the doctor do during them?*

A. The schedule of visits is often as follows:

- Every 4 weeks until 28 weeks
- Every 2 weeks from 30 to 36 weeks
- Weekly until delivery after 36 weeks

The doctor will always:

- Check your urine
- Check your weight and blood pressure
- Measure the size of your uterus (fundal height)
- Listen for fetal heart tones
- Educate and answer questions
- Perform special screening tests
- After 30 weeks, examine for the position of the fetus

TESTS

Q. *What does the CBC (complete blood count) tell us?*

A. It measures the number of red blood cells (RBCs) in your body, along with your hemoglobin (the oxygen-carrying protein found in the RBCs) and hematocrit (the percentage of RBCs relative to plasma—the fluid that allows the RBCs to flow in your vessels). If these are low, you are anemic and require treatment with iron. The number of white blood cells and platelets is also recorded.

Q. *What is the VDRL?*

A. This is a screening test for syphilis. Syphilis during pregnancy can cause a myriad of congenital anomalies in your fetus unless the disease is treated early in pregnancy.

Q. *What is the rubella test?*

A. Rubella is German measles. This test tells us if you are immune to the virus that causes German measles. This virus can cause many abnormalities in your fetus. If you are immune to the virus, you do not have to worry if you are exposed to it. If you are not immune to rubella, this test serves two purposes: First, if you are exposed to German measles, another rubella test can be drawn to verify whether you were actually infected. Second, a rubella vaccine will be given postpartum as an immunization for further pregnancies.

Q. *Why are the blood type and Rh titer drawn?*

A. The Rh titer is the most important part of this test during early pregnancy. The Rh antigen is a small protein found on the RBCs. Rh-positive means this protein is present. A woman with Rh-negative blood will have further tests during the course of her pregnancy. These will be discussed later.

Q. *What is cystic fibrosis?*

A. This is an inherited disorder that can affect the lungs, intestines, and reproductive organs. Thick mucous secretions can clog the lungs, causing decreased lung function with wheezing, coughing, and frequent lung infections. Thick mucus in the intestines causes diarrhea, abdominal pain, and poor weight gain and growth. Thick mucus in the reproductive tract can cause infertility. Life expectancy is less than normal in these individuals.

Q. *What happens if I am positive for the cystic fibrosis gene?*

A. Cystic fibrosis carriers are fairly common and unaffected by this recessive gene. Your partner will also be tested. If your partner is negative, there is nothing more to do during this pregnancy or any pregnancy with the same partner. If your partner is also a carrier, your baby has a 25 percent chance of having cystic fibrosis. If you want to know if your baby has cystic fibrosis, chorionic villus sampling (CVS) or amniocentesis can be performed.

Q. *What other screening tests might be performed?*

A. First-trimester screening for nuchal translucency with blood tests, alpha-fetoprotein quadruple screen, amniocentesis, chorionic villus sampling, diabetes screening, ultrasound, and another CBC and Rh titer (if you are Rh-negative) may be performed later in your pregnancy.

PREPARING FOR CHILDBIRTH

Q. *Should I take a childbirth class?*

A. If this is your first pregnancy, yes! There are many benefits to attending a childbirth class. Foremost is the psychological preparation for the pain of labor. If you know what to expect, you will deal with the pain of uterine contractions much more effectively. Women who take a childbirth class require less pain medication, and less often, during labor. Of course, you do not have to take these classes just to avoid pain medication during labor. You may take classes with the thought of having an epidural throughout labor. These classes also review the anatomy of the female reproductive system, the physiology and mechanics of labor, nutrition during pregnancy and postpartum, breast-feeding, cesarean sections, fetal monitoring, and hospital procedures. There are two schools of prepared childbirth—Lamaze and Bradley.

Q. *What is the Lamaze method?*

A. The Lamaze method, or the psychoprophylactic method (PPM), relies on the principle of conditioning against pain. By practicing relaxation techniques, the woman will be able to concentrate on relieving tension when a labor contraction (pain) occurs. This is done, with the help of her partner, by utilizing different breathing patterns during labor. It is often a rewarding team effort, in which couples successfully work together through each contraction.

Q. *What is the Bradley method?*

A. The Bradley method is a stricter form of childbirth that emphasizes a "natural" birth with the avoidance of any medication for pain. This method teaches women to concentrate on the pain instead of avoiding it by using breathing patterns. Several methods of relaxation are taught, and women are encouraged to use the method that best suits them. The partner acts as a support person who encourages the woman during labor with positive statements. This method also recommends that the couple create their own unique birth plan for labor and delivery and discuss it with their doctor.

Q. *What is a doula?*

A. The doula (from the Greek, meaning "in service of") provides physical and emotional support for the laboring woman and her partner during childbirth but does not assess the mother's or fetus's well-being. The monitrice (from the French, meaning "to watch over attentively") is a nurse whose role is the same as a doula's but in addition may do clinical assessment on mother and fetus. Studies have shown that birth advocates have had a positive influence on the outcome of labor and deliveries.

Q. *How are childbirth classes offered?*

A. The classes are offered once a week for 3 to 8 weeks. Each class is about 3 hours long.

Q. *When do I take these classes?*

A. Plan on beginning the class at about your 30th week so that you can finish the classes before you deliver. Also, you should have plenty of time to practice what you have learned in class.

Q. *Are there warning signs that I should be aware of and notify my doctor about?*

A. There are several complications of pregnancy that may occur. Fortunately, most pregnancies progress without difficulty. However, call your doctor immediately if you experience any of these symptoms:

- Vaginal spotting not related to intercourse
- Vaginal bleeding
- A gush of fluid or a steady flow of fluid from your vagina
- Continuous vomiting
- Frequent and painful urination
- Fever (over 100.4°F) and chills with flank pain or abdominal pain not accompanied by diarrhea or the flu
- Labor contractions lasting at least 45 seconds and occurring fewer than 10 minutes apart before your 37th week of pregnancy
- Severe persistent headache
- Blurred vision
- Sudden swelling in your hands and face
- Sudden and rapid weight gain
- Decreased urination despite normal or increased drinking habits
- Right upper abdominal pain
- Decreased or absent fetal movement for 24 hours in the third trimester

CHAPTER 2

Growth and
Development of the Fetus

Q. *How long does the average pregnancy last?*

A. The average pregnancy, or gestation, lasts 280 days, or 40 weeks, or ten lunar (4-week) months, or nine calendar months. Obstetricians calculate the pregnancy from the first day of your last menstrual period (LMP).

Ovulation and conception, however, do not occur until 14 days later, so the fetus grows for about 266 days. Your pregnancy is also divided into three equal trimesters. The duration of each trimester is 13 weeks, or three calendar months.

Q. *How do you calculate the delivery date?*

A. You may calculate the delivery date by using Nägele's rule: subtract three months from your LMP and add 7 days. For example, if your LMP was December 22, your due date would be September 29. The EDC (estimated date of confinement) is your due date. Your doctor will have a pregnancy wheel or calculator to calculate your EDC. Calculation of the due date is based on a 28-day menstrual cycle with ovulation occurring on the 14th day. If your menstrual cycle is longer or shorter than 28 days, you must add (if longer) or subtract (if shorter) the corresponding number of days.

Q. *What are the chances of delivering on the EDC?*

A. About 5 percent of women will have their delivery on the EDC. About 50 percent will deliver within 1 week, and 85 percent will deliver within 2 weeks before or after the EDC.

Q. *When does the fetus first move?*

A. It has been shown, using ultrasound, that the fetus twitches between 7 and 10 weeks, moves arms and legs at 10 to 12 weeks, and moves limbs, head, and torso by 16 weeks.

Q. *When will I first feel my baby move?*

A. Usually between 16 and 20 weeks, you may notice a slight fluttering in your abdomen that will become increasingly strong as the days go by. The first feeling of fetal activity is called "quickening" and is your first perception that your fetus is alive. If this is your first pregnancy, expect to feel fetal movement at or after 20 weeks and even later if your placenta is anterior (located on the belly side of the uterus). Multiparous women (those who have had multiple prior births) may feel fetal movement as early as 15 weeks.

Q. *What is the placenta?*

A. The placenta is an organ of the fetus that serves many functions. It attaches to your uterus and is bathed by your blood, taking oxygen and nutrients to the fetus and returning fetal waste products back into your circulation for disposal. The placenta can also actively transport certain substances from your blood to the fetus, such as proteins and calcium, which are needed in greater amounts for growth. Almost anything that gets into your circulation can get into the fetal bloodstream, including medications and drugs, if the molecules are small enough. Viruses can also pass through the placenta, but the placenta actively transports your antibodies to the fetus to provide immunity against disease. The placenta also produces several different hormones that maintain and increase the growth of the fetus. One of these hormones is called human chorionic gonadotropin (HCG); this is the hormone measured in pregnancy tests.

Q. *What is the umbilical cord?*

A. The umbilical cord is the lifeline for your fetus. The umbilical cord attaches from the placenta to the umbilicus (navel, or belly button) of the fetus. The umbilical cord contains three vessels—two arteries and one vein. The umbilical vein carries oxygenated and nutrient-rich blood from the placenta to the fetus, and the umbilical arteries carry oxygen-poor blood back to the placenta. These vessels are cushioned by a substance called Wharton's jelly and are all wrapped by amniotic membrane. At birth, the average length of the umbilical cord is about 21 inches, with a normal range of 12 to 42 inches. The width is about 1 inch.

Q. *What happens during the first month of pregnancy?*

A. Remember that you do not become pregnant until after ovulation, which takes place on about day 14 of a 28-day menstrual cycle. Fertilization of your egg by your partner's sperm follows on that day. During the next 6 days, the fertilized egg, or zygote, travels down your fallopian tube and divides into sixteen cells (the morula) by day 17 and into the many-celled blastocyst by day 20. The blastocyst attaches to your uterus on day 20 or 21 of your cycle, or 6 to 7 days after ovulation. This is called implantation. On the 22nd day, the blastocyst separates into what will become the placenta and your baby, called the trophoblast and embryo, respectively. On day 26, the circulation between your uterus and the placenta has been established and the amniotic cavity has formed. On day 28, the 14-day-old embryo is composed of three different cell layers and has formed the chorioamniotic sac. The pregnancy is now completely surrounded by specialized uterine tissue called decidua. The embryo is about 2 millimeters, or ½ of an inch, long.

Q. *How does my baby develop throughout pregnancy (after day 1 of my last menstrual period)?*

A. *At 6 weeks,* the embryo's chin rests on its chest, and limb buds have formed. There is a prominent tail. The heart has started beating by 5 weeks, and by the end of 6 weeks, it has four chambers. The beginnings of the brain and spinal cord have formed. In fact, all major organs have begun to form. The embryo is now floating in amniotic fluid and may be seen by ultrasound.

At 8 weeks, the fetus is about one-half head, and you can see its eyes, ears, nose, and mouth. The intestines are in the umbilical cord. The fingers and toes have formed, and the tail has almost disappeared. Your uterus is about the size of an orange.

At 12 weeks, the fingers have started growing nails. The arms and legs can now bend and have reached their relative length in comparison to the rest of the body. The intestines are now back in the abdomen. The face has become more human looking. There are about 1½ ounces of amniotic fluid. Your uterus is about the size of a cantaloupe.

At 16 weeks, you can now see a rudimentary penis or vagina. Scalp hair has begun to form, and your fetus is actively moving about. It has breathing movements and has begun to swallow amniotic fluid. The fetus also starts urinating now. Bones have started to form. The top of your uterus, called the fundus, can be felt midway between your pubic bone and belly button. There are about 8 ounces of amniotic fluid. The fetus may start sucking its thumb.

At 20 weeks, vernix caseosa, a white cheesy material composed of oil and old fetal skin cells, covers the fetus, protecting its skin from becoming macerated (soft and flaky) by the amniotic fluid. The toenails begin to develop. The face is fully developed now. There are about 13 ounces of amniotic fluid.

At 24 weeks, the skin is wrinkled and has very delicate hair called lanugo growing all over its body. Eyebrows and eyelashes appear now, too. Fat starts developing. Breathing movements are more regular, but the lungs are not well developed. If birth occurs now, survival is rare but possible.

At 28 weeks, the skin is now red and shiny and has lost its wrinkles owing to the deposition of more fat. But the body is still lean and trim. The eyelids have opened now. Your fetus may appear to move less, but that's just because there is more room for it to move around. If birth occurs now, chance of survival is good and better with every day (thanks to technology).

At 32 weeks, your fetus is about 16 inches long and weighs 3¾ pounds. If the baby is born prematurely now, his or her chance of surviving is over 90 percent.

At 36 weeks, the body is now plump, and the lanugo hairs have begun to disappear. The fingernails and toenails reach to the tips. The skin is pink and smooth. If a male, the testes have begun to descend into the scrotum.

At 40 weeks, the average length is 19½ inches, and your baby may weigh from 6 to 10 pounds or more. The average weight is 7½ pounds.

CHAPTER 3

Common Complaints During Pregnancy

Q. *Why do I urinate so frequently at the beginning and end of my pregnancy?*

A. First, we must understand the anatomy of the bladder and its relationship to the uterus. The bladder rests on top of the uterus. In the first trimester, as the uterus grows, the bladder is stretched. A woman's brain perceives this signal as the sensation of a full bladder. In addition, the rate of urine production is increased.

You may also notice a decrease in the frequency of urination in the middle of your pregnancy and then an increase again after 32 weeks, due to the increased pressure on the bladder by the growing head of the fetus.

Q. *Is it common to leak urine when I cough, laugh, sneeze, jump, or run during pregnancy?*

A. Yes, this is very common and is due to the changing position of the bladder throughout pregnancy. Kegel exercises may decrease the frequency of this sometimes embarrassing condition. This annoyance usually disappears a few months postpartum.

Q. *Is it common to lose urine*
   spontaneously during my pregnancy?

A. Yes. Spontaneous loss of urine while awake or asleep is common, especially in the late second trimester and third trimester. Leaking urine is more common with each subsequent pregnancy.

Q. *How can I tell if I accidentally*
   urinated or if I ruptured my bag of water?

A. Sometimes you can't. The fluid may not smell like urine or amniotic fluid. Usually, after you break your membranes you will leak continuously or intermittently, but not always. Therefore, you must get checked if you are not sure. Place your wet panties in a plastic bag and bring it to your doctor's office or L&D to be checked. You will also be examined to determine if the fluid was urine or amniotic fluid.

Q. *What are Kegel exercises?*

A. Kegel exercises are designed to strengthen the muscles of your pelvic floor to gain better control of your bladder both during pregnancy and postpartum. To do these exercises, contract and loosen the muscles around your vagina, much like you would if you were starting and stopping the flow of urine during urination (you may practice this while urinating, too). Hold each contraction to a count of ten. Do sets of ten or twenty each day. (You can do this exercise in the car while waiting at a red light or during a commercial break while watching TV.)

A variant of the Kegel exercises is contracting and holding the muscle of your rectal sphincter (as when you do not want to pass gas in public), which some believe will decrease the incidence of vaginal lacerations or episiotomies. This exercise will certainly increase the tone of your pelvic floor muscles.

Q. *In early pregnancy, is mild uterine cramping normal?*

A. Yes, it is. This cramping is called *Braxton Hicks contractions* and can be mildly uncomfortable. This cramping can begin as early as 8 weeks. If the cramps are severe or accompanied by vaginal bleeding, contact your obstetrician.

Q. *Are Braxton Hicks contractions common?*

A. Yes. Usually you will feel this tightening of your uterus beginning in the second trimester. They can feel sharp for 5 seconds or feel like a dull and mild menstrual cramp for up to 30 seconds. Near the end of the third trimester, you may confuse Braxton Hicks contractions with early labor.

Other facts about Braxton Hicks contractions:

- You may not experience these contractions.
- They can be more intense with each pregnancy. You may feel more intense pains, although they are still mild.
- If you had them with your first pregnancy, you may not have them with the second.
- If you have a lot of them during your third trimester, that doesn't mean you will have your baby early.
- Braxton Hicks contractions have nothing to do with when you will go into labor.

Q. *What do I do when I have a*
Braxton Hicks contraction?

A. Ignore it. If they become frequent, change your activity. If you are walking, sit or lie down. I discuss false labor in Chapter 10.

Q. *In early pregnancy, is it normal to have*
pains going down to the groin?

A. Yes. This is called the *round ligament syndrome*. These ligaments attach from the top of the uterus to your groin area. The pain you feel may be sharp or dull and may be felt on both sides or only one side of your lower abdomen or groin. The pain may be intensified by movement. You may get some relief by going into the knee-chest position by bringing your knees up to your chest.

Q. *In mid- to late pregnancy, is it*
common to experience a pain that
shoots up the midline of my belly and
also down the insides of my thighs?

A. Yes. This pain, called *symphysis pubis* pain, is due to the separation of the pubic bones. Relaxin, another placental hormone, relaxes the fibers connecting the bones. The movement of these bones is perceived as pain over your pubic region and inner thighs. This discomfort can range from mildly annoying to severe. The pain is intensified by walking, especially up stairs, and may even be felt in the sitting position. You will notice that you will walk in a crab- or duck-like waddle to decrease the pain. Sometimes your first episode of symphysis pubis pain will occur after vaginal delivery and stretching of these fibers. This pain will disappear by the third postpartum month.

Q. *Is back pain common during pregnancy?*

A. Yes. About half of pregnant moms will experience back pain, usually occurring in the late second to third trimester. This pain can linger into your sixth postpartum month.

Q. *Who gets back pain during pregnancy?*

A. The only risk factor for back pain during pregnancy is prior back pain and previous full-term pregnancies. Age, your weight, fetal weight, or multiple pregnancies do not increase the incidence of back pain.

Q. *What causes back pain during pregnancy?*

A. Your enlarging uterus changes your posture. Your abdominal muscles become stretched and weakened, which decreases their ability to maintain proper posture. This puts added strain on your back muscles, which tire, spasm, and hurt. Relaxin, the placental hormone that causes joint laxity, weakens support of the spine and pelvic bones. This causes movement and stretching of nerve fibers, which are perceived as pain.

Q. *What types of back pain could I get during pregnancy?*

A. There are three types of back pain you could experience during pregnancy: lumbar pain, nocturnal back pain, and sacroiliac pain.

Q. *What is lumbar pain?*

A. Lumbar pain is characterized by pain located in the middle of your lower back. The pain may also radiate, or travel, down the back of one or both of your legs. Lumbar pain is worse when standing or sitting. As your pregnancy progresses, the size and weight of the uterus changes your center of balance. To compensate for this change, your posture changes: you lean backward, making the lower muscles in your back work harder, causing muscle strain.

Q. *How can I prevent lumbar pain*
during pregnancy?

A. To prevent lumbar pain during pregnancy, begin exercising prior to your pregnancy. Women who work out experience less lumbar pain during pregnancy. They have strengthened the back muscles needed to maintain proper posture throughout their pregnancy. Prolonged standing or sitting may increase the incidence and severity of lumbar pain. Placing one foot on a small footstool will tilt your pelvis forward and decrease strain on your lumbar spine and muscles. Wearing shoes with low heels will decrease pain as well.

Q. *What is the treatment for lumbar pain?*

A. Heat or cold to the back is safe and may relieve your symptoms. You may use both a heating pad and a cold pack. The heat is soothing. Ice will numb the pain. Acetaminophen may be used. A TENS (transcutaneous electrical nerve stimulation) unit may be used. Sleep on a firm mattress. Sit on a straight-back chair, and try not to slouch on a couch. When bending down, bend from your knees, not from your waist. A maternity girdle may be useful, especially if you have poor abdominal muscle tone. Try to maintain an erect posture. You can try to improve your posture by standing next to a wall, making sure your head, shoulders, back, and buttocks are touching the wall at the same time for 5 to 10 seconds five to ten times a day. If your pain persists, see a physical therapist. An exercise regimen prescribed by a certified physical therapist can be beneficial. The physical therapist will also observe your posture while you are standing and teach you how to maintain a proper posture, which should decrease your pain. Whirlpool baths, joint manipulation, ibuprofen, and muscle relaxants are not appropriate treatments during pregnancy. Massage therapy, however, may provide short-term relief.

Q. *What is nocturnal back pain?*

A. This is back pain that occurs only while lying down at night. This pain is caused by the swelling of tissues in your back. This edema (excess fluid in tissues) pushes and pinches nerves, causing back pain.

Q. *What is sacroiliac pain?*

A. This is pain caused by movement of this joint, which stretches pain-sensitive structures. This joint is normally stable and nonmoving. The joint is made up of your tailbone and pelvic bone. The movement is enabled by relaxin, a placental hormone, which relaxes the joint, causing the pain. Sacroiliac pain is four times more common than lumbar pain.

Q. *What are the characteristics of*
   sacroiliac pain?

A. You may experience pain in one or both buttocks. The pain may or may not radiate or travel down to the back of your mid thigh.

Q. *What is the treatment for sacroiliac pain?*

A. Heat may be soothing. Ice can be beneficial for its numbing effect. A nonelastic trochanteric belt fit by a physical therapist may decrease pain with walking. A physical therapist may also prescribe exercises to reduce the intensity of your pain. Unfortunately, prepregnancy fitness will not prevent sacroiliac pain during pregnancy.

Q. *Why do I have upper back pain?*

A. You may experience upper back pain stemming from your change in posture. The muscles in your upper back must adjust and are sore. The upper back muscles will also have to support your enlarging breasts. Their heavy weight will pull on these muscles as well.

Q. *What can I do to relieve upper back pain?*

A. Wear a support bra, see a physical therapist and a massage therapist, and start exercises to increase the strength of your upper back muscles.

Q. *Why are my breasts tender?*

A. The increase in the production of estrogen causes the breast tissue to swell and become tender. This tenderness is usually most annoying during the first 6 to 12 weeks of your pregnancy.

Q. *When will my breasts begin to grow?*

A. Beginning at 6 weeks, your breasts will begin to enlarge as a result of water retention in the breast tissue. After 8 weeks, the milk glands and ducts begin to enlarge along with the increased growth of fatty tissue.

Q. *What other changes will occur in my breasts?*

A. Because of the increase in breast tissue, there will be an increase in blood supply. You may notice the appearance of bluish veins in the skin on your breasts. Your areolas and nipples will darken. The nipples will become much larger and erectile to accommodate feeding your baby. If there is a great increase in the size of your breasts, you may develop stretch marks.

Q. *How big will my breasts grow?*

A. Every woman is different, but expect at least a two-cup change and a ½-pound increase in the weight of each breast.

Q. *What is colostrum?*

A. Colostrum is a thick, yellowish fluid discharged from the breast. Colostrum may appear anytime after the first trimester, with its quantity increasing after delivery. Colostrum nourishes the baby before your milk comes in. It also contains antibodies that will provide your baby with immunity to diseases to which you have resistance.

Q. *What should I do to prevent or treat caked nipples?*

A. Caked nipples are caused by colostrum that has dried on your nipples. If you are leaking colostrum, place a cotton or gauze pad into your bra to absorb the fluid. If your nipples are already caked with dried colostrum, wash your breasts with warm water only, two or three times a day. You can use a breast cream or lanolin to combat dryness and cracking.

Q. *What causes constipation during pregnancy?*

A. Constipation occurs in about 30 percent of pregnant women during the first and third trimesters. Decreased intestinal motion and/or increased absorption of water by the intestine, caused by an increase in the hormone progesterone, can cause constipation and harder stools. Iron found in your prenatal vitamins may also cause constipation. Moreover, your enlarging uterus may press down on your large intestine and cause a slowdown.

Q. *What can I do to prevent or relieve constipation?*

A. To prevent or relieve constipation, try the following:

- Drink at least eight glasses of fluids a day.
- Eat vegetables, fruits, and bran.
- Increase your physical activity.
- Ask your doctor if you could use a laxative such as milk of magnesia, Senekot, or Colace or Metamucil.
- Avoid foods such as bananas, rice, apples, or toast (this is the BRAT diet used if you have diarrhea!).

Q. *What causes leg cramps?*

A. Leg cramps occur after the first trimester, becoming more common until the last month of pregnancy, when they occur infrequently. They are most likely to occur at night when you are sleeping or lying down. Either too little calcium or too much phosphorus in your diet can cause them. Calcium is found in milk and cheese, as is phosphorus. Phosphorus is also found in red meat. Or you may be absorbing calcium poorly. Inactivity and weight gain can cause leg cramps. Poor circulation and your enlarging uterus will cause pressure on the nerves and blood vessels going to your legs, which can also cause leg cramps.

Q. *What can I do to prevent leg cramps?*

A. To prevent leg cramps, try the following:

- Drink no more than 1 pint of milk a day.
- Limit the amount of red meat in your diet to one serving a day.
- Supplement your diet with 1 to 2 grams of magnesium oxide pills.
- Stretch your legs for 30 seconds each night before going to sleep.
- Raise the foot of your bed 6 inches.
- Sleep on your side, not on your back.
- Wear support hose or socks.

You can take acetaminophen if the pain from a leg cramp is persistent and annoying. Call your physician if your leg cramps become more frequent and more painful.

Q. *What can I do when I get a leg cramp?*

A. Turn over on your side or stand up to increase circulation to your legs. Point your foot toward your face to stretch the calf muscle. Rub and/or apply heat to your calf.

Q. *What is Restless Leg Syndrome (RLS)?*

A. RLS is a common neurological disorder. You may have a very unpleasant feeling in your legs that is relieved by moving your legs. These sensations have been described as itching, tingling, twitching, prickly, pins and needles, crawling, or pulling. Moving your legs make them feel better but only temporarily. RLS symptoms are worse at bedtime.

RLS is more common during pregnancy. Up to 27 percent of pregnant women may develop RLS. The symptoms can become increasingly common and bothersome in the third trimester. We don't know what the cause is, but we do know that the development of RLS during pregnancy is temporary and will disappear postpartum.

Q. *What is the treatment for RLS during pregnancy?*

A. Try the following:

- If you are anemic as a result of a folic acid or iron deficiency, replacement therapy may help.
- Do not exercise close to your bedtime.
- Leg massage and cold compresses may relieve symptoms.
- Try going to bed and waking up at the same time every day.
- Ultimately, delivery cures almost all RLS that develops during pregnancy.

Q. *Why did I become dizzy when I got out of bed this morning?*

A. During pregnancy, your blood pressure may be lower than normal owing to hormonal changes that cause your blood vessels to dilate. The vessels do not constrict as quickly or as efficiently in response to a change in your position. Therefore, standing up too fast doesn't allow your circulatory system to adjust in time, not enough blood and oxygen reach your brain, and you feel faint. In addition, you may be anemic, so the oxygen-carrying capacity of your blood will be reduced; and after an overnight fast, low blood sugar may compound this problem. Dizziness is more common in women with varicose veins. You may also experience dizziness later in pregnancy if you lie on your back because your heavy uterus presses on the vena cava (the large vein that brings blood to your heart), decreasing the blood return.

Q. *What can I do to prevent this dizziness?*

A. Inform your doctor, who may want to test you for anemia and prescribe iron therapy. When getting out of bed, sit up and wait 15 seconds, then hang your legs off the bed and wait 15 seconds, then stand and wait 15 seconds, and then start walking. If you notice that dizziness during the day is relieved by a snack, drink a glass of orange juice before getting out of bed.

Standing in place and not moving allows your blood to pool in your legs and can also make you dizzy. To avoid this, walk in place; your calf muscles will help pump your blood back to your heart. Taking a hot shower and standing in place as you shampoo your hair is a high-risk combination for dizziness and fainting.

Q. *Is it normal to be tired all the time?*
What causes this fatigue?

A. Yes, it may begin in the first trimester and linger throughout your pregnancy. The increased level of progesterone produces a sedative effect. Fatigue is also one of the characteristic signs of anemia.

Q. *What should I do about fatigue?*

A. Tell your doctor, who will probably test you for anemia. If you are anemic, iron therapy will be prescribed. You will feel better in about 5 weeks. If you are not anemic, then you need more rest; go to sleep earlier and, if you can, take a nap or lie down during the day.

Q. *Is memory loss common during pregnancy?*

A. Pregnesia, or loss of memory during pregnancy, is a common occurrence. It is due to the hormones of pregnancy. This condition may last throughout your pregnancy and for a few months postpartum. This "brain drain" is never complete, is variable among women, and may change throughout your pregnancy.

Q. *Are mood swings common in pregnancy?*
What causes them?

A. They sure are. Almost every pregnant woman will experience at least one or two episodes of mood swings, most commonly during the first and third trimesters.

Pregnancy is a life-changing event. Any major change in one's life can cause stress. Even a happy event, an anticipated event, or a planned event can cause stress and mood swings. Although you are overcome with joy about being pregnant, you may still worry about miscarriage, birth defects, the health of your growing baby, your delivery, your parenting abilities, your changing relationship with your partner and other children, and finances. On top of this add the large influx of pregnancy hormones into your system, which can cause fatigue, irritability, sleep disturbances, and nausea and other unpleasant side effects. This can all blunt your ability to cope with day-to-day activities and contribute to the frequency of mood swings.

Q. *How can I cope with mood swings?*

A. You must remember that mood swings commonly occur during pregnancy:

- Warn your partner.
- Exercise; the endorphins that are released in your brain will make you feel better.
- If you are extremely fatigued, try to get plenty of sleep at night. Find a way to nap during the day.
- Spend time relaxing with your favorite hobby. Watch comedies and read humorous books. Meditate. Get a massage. Spend a day at a spa.

Q. *When are mood swings serious?*

A. If your mood swings are lasting all day long and are interfering with your daily life, consult your doctor. For example, if you do not want to get out of bed in the morning despite a restful night's sleep; if you have stopped eating, although you are not nauseous; if you can't concentrate at work; or if you can't fall asleep at night because of your to anxiety, call your doctor. You do not have mood swings. You have depression.

Q. *Is flatulence (gas) more common during pregnancy?*

A. Yes. Both flatulence and belching can increase during pregnancy. Intestinal gas will cause your abdomen to distend, and you may feel bloated. To minimize these feelings, avoid foods such as cabbage and beans. Simethicone can be used to relieve the symptoms of excess gas. It works by breaking up gas bubbles in your digestive tract. Simethicone does not get absorbed into your bloodstream and is safe to use if needed.

Q. *Can pregnancy cause my gums*
to bleed and swell?

A. Yes. This is called pregnancy gingivitis, and it occurs in at least 30 percent of pregnant women. It can begin as early as the first month of pregnancy and can become progressively worse. Your gums will return to their normal state one to two months after delivery.

Q. *What causes pregnancy gingivitis?*

A. An increase in estrogen and progesterone causes an increase in blood flow and blood vessels to your to gums, which causes swelling. These hormonal changes also decrease your mouth's ability to combat the bacteria that cause gum disease, or peridontitis. Pregnancy gingivitis starts in the first trimester and worsens throughout your pregnancy.

Q. *Can pregnancy gingivitis be prevented?*

A. Not always, but the severity can be minimized with the use of a toothbrush and dental floss. Begin good oral hygiene early. Get your dental checkup before your pregnancy. Maintain your oral hygiene by having regular teeth cleaning by your dentist or oral hygienist throughout your pregnancy. Pregnancy gingivitis is only a pregnancy complication. The swelling, bleeding, and gum sensitivity will disappear during the postpartum period. If these symptoms persist, you have periodontal disease and should consult your dentist.

Q. *Can I grow hair in abnormal places during my pregnancy?*

A. Yes. Many women will notice the increased growth of fine hairs on their face, arms, and legs. Occasionally, new pubic hair will grow in the midline of your lower abdomen up toward your navel.

Q. *Will these hairs disappear?*

A. Yes. Usually in two to six months following delivery, these hairs will disappear, but they can return with each new pregnancy.

Q. *How are headaches treated during pregnancy?*

A. Headaches may occur throughout your pregnancy. The possible causes are numerous—emotional tension, sinusitis, eyestrain, fatigue, and anemia. Conservative therapy is always the initial step. Try lying down in a dark room and relaxing. A cold or hot compress may provide relief. Acetaminophen (Tylenol) or aspirin may be used during pregnancy, but ask your doctor first before self-prescribing medications.

Q. *Sometimes I feel my heart pounding. How come?*

A. This is a common disturbance during the last trimester. It is due to the increased blood volume and increased work performed by your heart. If the problem becomes frequent, tell your doctor. When it occurs, sit or lie down and relax; the episode usually lasts only a few seconds.

Q. *How common is heartburn*
    during pregnancy?

A. It affects up to 75 percent of pregnant women, usually beginning in the second trimester and becoming more frequent thereafter.
About 25 percent of these women will experience it every day. The
medical term for heartburn is gastrointestinal esophageal reflux disease, or GERD. Your esophagus, which is the tube from your mouth
to your stomach, feels like it is burning—not your heart.

Q. *What causes heartburn*
    during pregnancy?

A. The increase in progesterone causes the stomach to empty into
the intestines at a slower rate and also relaxes the valve between the
stomach and esophagus, allowing acid to enter the esophagus. As
the pregnant uterus grows, it pushes into the stomach, giving it less
space and increasing the frequency of your symptoms.

Q. *How can I decrease the frequency of*
    heartburn or control its symptoms?

A. To lesson the frequency of heartburn, eat several small meals
during the day instead of three big meals. After meals, sit or walk;
don't lie down. Drink milk or eat some yogurt. You can also try
sleeping on your side; but if you prefer to sleep on your back, try
propping up your head and back with several pillows.

Antacids are the treatment of choice for heartburn during pregnancy. Avoid preparations that contain sodium, which can lead to uncomfortable water retention. Antacids may be taken 1 hour before
and 2 hours after meals and at bedtime. I suggest using antacids that

contain both calcium and magnesium; the magnesium will decrease your risk of constipation. Antacids that contain only calcium or calcium and aluminum can increase your chances of constipation.

If your GERD is 24/7, consult your doctor about using a long-acting medicine that blocks the secretion of acid from your stomach. These meds, such as Zantac or Pepsid, are safe to take during pregnancy, and you will be able to sleep throughout the night symptom free.

Q. *Why do pregnant women develop hemorrhoids (piles)?*

A. Hemorrhoids are distended vessels or varicose veins located in the anus. They are caused by a combination of the increased blood volume and growing weight of the pregnant uterus on the great vessels. Hemorrhoids appear to be hereditary. They usually appear in the third trimester or during the second stage of labor, as a consequence of your pushing efforts.

Q. *Are hemorrhoids dangerous?*

A. No, just uncomfortable and annoying. Hemorrhoids make their appearance known by causing rectal pain, itching, swelling, and/or bleeding. The bleeding can range from spotting to a large amount, which stops on its own. If you are unsure of the source of your bleeding, rectal or vaginal, contact your doctor.

Q. *How can I prevent and treat hemorrhoids?*

A. To prevent hemorrhoids, avoid constipation and hard stools. If you feel the urge to defecate, do not delay. Eat a high-fiber diet and drink lots of fluid.

Replace all hemorrhoids protruding out of your anus with gentle finger pressure as soon as you discover them. Hot sitz baths two or three times a day may be soothing. Witch hazel or lemon juice may decrease swelling. Over-the-counter hemorrhoid preparations may be used in the second and third trimesters after consulting your doctor.

Q. *When is the most common time for nausea and vomiting (morning sickness) to occur?*

A. Up to 85 percent of pregnant women will experience nausea and/or vomiting and not necessarily in the morning. Symptoms usually begin by your 6th week but may appear as late as your 9th week. If you experience nausea and vomiting after your 9th week, check with your doctor; some other condition besides pregnancy may be causing your symptoms.

Morning sickness is just a general term for nausea and vomiting during pregnancy because it is usually most common and annoying in the morning for most pregnant women. Some women, however, are never nauseous in the morning but are nauseous the rest of the day or only in the evenings.

Q. *Are there risk factors that make me more susceptible to morning sickness?*

A. Yes. If you felt nauseous on birth control pills, you have a good chance of being nauseous during pregnancy. A past history of nausea in a prior pregnancy puts you at risk for more of the same in subsequent pregnancies—a 68 percent risk if symptoms were severe and a 50 percent risk if they were mild. If your mom or sister had morning sickness, so may you. Female fetus may increase your risk. Multiple fetuses increase your risk because of multiple placentas. If you tend to have migraine headaches or experience motion sickness, your risk for nausea and vomiting is increased.

Q. *What can I do to relieve my nausea?*

A. Nausea occurs most commonly on an empty stomach. Since you are not eating while you sleep, nausea is most common in the morning—hence the name morning sickness. You can't prevent nausea, but taking a multivitamin before pregnancy may decrease the severity of nausea during pregnancy.

To relieve nausea, try to eat small, frequent meals throughout the day and try to eat your meals slowly. Before you go to sleep at night, eat a slice of turkey, chicken, or cheese. These high-protein foods are digested more slowly, keeping food in your stomach for a longer period of time. In the morning before you get out of bed, eat two or three crackers with some milk and then remain in bed for another 10 to 15 minutes. Also, you may want to avoid certain foods that are greasy and spicy. Nausea may be caused by your body reacting to the hormones of pregnancy or too little glycogen—a sugar stored in your liver. Ice-cold fluids sipped through a straw from a sealed container will avoid taste and smell triggers that cause nausea. Stop taking your prenatal vitamins for a few days—this may relieve some of your nausea.

There are several nonprescription and prescription medications that may work for you:

- Motion sickness wrist bands are effective in 10 to 15 percent of cases.
- Take vitamin B_6, 10 to 25 milligrams every 6 hours.
- Doxylamine, which can help relieve nausea, can be found in nonprescription sleeping pills. You can take

it at night, or you can take ½ tablet every 6 hours along with 25 milligrams of vitamin B_6.

- If you are still nauseous, you can add dimenhydrinate, 50 to 100 milligrams every 4 to 6 hours. Use up to 400 milligrams a day if used alone or 200 milligrams a day if used with doxylamine.
- Emmetrol is an over-the-counter (OTC) sugary syrup used to control nausea.
- Fresh ginger is fine to use, but avoid ginger capsules, which may thin your blood and decrease platelet function.

Q. *I am still really nauseous and vomiting. Now what should I do?*

A. If your nausea and vomiting is still not under sufficient control after trying nonprescription methods or if these medicines are giving you undesirable side effects, it is time to try or add prescription medicines. Every doctor has a favorite regimen or first choice of meds to use. I start with metoclopramide, 5 to10 milligrams every 6 to 8 hours as needed. This drug increases the contractions of your stomach and intestines. So besides treating your nausea and vomiting, it will also lessen your heartburn. In addition, if you take it at bedtime, you will wake up the next morning without feeling like you have a bag of acid in your belly. Phenothiazine medications can be taken orally or rectally. These meds can be added to any regimen. Ondansetron 8-milligram melts can be cut in half and used every 4 hours as needed. This medicine is very expensive, even with prescription coverage. The major side effect is constipation with hard stools, so use a stool softener.

Q. *What is hyperemesis gravidarum?*

A. Hyperemesis gravidarum is nausea and vomiting that is so severe, continuous, and unrelenting that it causes severe weight loss,
dehydration, and salt disturbances. Luckily, this condition occurs
in less than 1 percent of pregnancies.

Q. *What is the treatment of*
hyperemesis gravidarum?

A. The initial treatment will involve hospitalization with IV fluid
replacement and medications. If stabilization is quick, you may be
discharged with your IV and treated by a home health care nurse
under your doctor's supervision. If your symptoms persist and you
are unable to tolerate food or water, eventually you may require
tube feedings or IV nutrition. This will provide the necessary calories, proteins, and essential fats that your body has been using up
by breaking down your fat and muscles. Hyperemesis gravidarum
usually lasts until the end of the first trimester, rarely lasting up to
the 18th week.

Q. *I've had a stuffy nose ever since I became*
pregnant. Did I develop an allergy?

A. Nasal stuffiness is common and is due to swollen mucous
membranes in the nasal passages. The swelling is caused by the increase in your blood circulation. You may also develop a chronic
cough from a postnasal drip.

Q. *How can I treat these symptoms?*

A. Using a humidifier may reduce the frequency and severity of these problems. A nasal decongestant may be used under your doctor's direction.

Q. *Are nosebleeds more common*
during pregnancy?

A. Yes. This is due to the increased number of new blood vessels in the mucous membranes of your nose and the increased circulation. The bleeding almost always stops on its own. When a nosebleed does occur, apply a cold compress to your nose. A humidifier may help prevent nosebleeds.

Q. *My fingernails keep breaking.*
What can I do to prevent this?

A. Changes in your nails may occur as early as the 6th week of your pregnancy. Brittle nails due to thinning and softening of your nails and accelerated growth of one's nails are common. A diet with adequate amounts of protein and calcium will help keep your nails hard. Keep your nails short if they continue to break. These nail changes are not permanent.

Q. *Why do my arms and hands feel numb,*
and why do my fingers tingle?

A. Stretching the nerves in your neck that supply your hands causes this condition, which affects 5 to 10 percent of pregnant women. It is due to drooping of your shoulders and affects both hands. Numbness is most common upon wakening in the morning and may persist after delivery because of the constant carrying of your baby.

Q. *How can I prevent this?*

A. Practice good posture (see questions on backaches earlier in this chapter).

Q. *Why do the lateral three fingers of my hand burn and have a pins-and-needles sensation?*

A. This is called *carpal tunnel syndrome* and usually affects only one hand. It is caused by compression of the median nerve by the swelling of tissues in the wrist. This condition is more common near the end of pregnancy and usually disappears postpartum.

Q. *What is the treatment for carpal tunnel syndrome?*

A. To treat carpal tunnel syndrome:

- Restrict your intake of salty foods.
- Raise your hands above your head when lying down.
- A wrist splint called a neutral splint can be prescribed by your doctor. If your pain persists, get a referral to a hand physical therapist.

Q. *Is it common to have shortness of breath or to hyperventilate?*

A. A feeling of "air hunger" or shortness of breath can occur anytime during pregnancy. The cause is twofold. In the first two trimesters, the added supply of progesterone increases the sensitivity of the respiratory center in the brain to carbon dioxide, causing a faster breathing rate. In the third trimester, your growing uterus presses into your lungs and crowds them.

Q. *How can I stop this feeling?*

A. Try the following:

- Raise your arms over your head.
- Sleep with several pillows under your head and back.
- Take long deep breaths and relax. Remember, this is a normal change during pregnancy.

Q. *What is the "mask of pregnancy"?*

A. This condition (also called *melasma* or *chloasma*), which occurs in at least 70 percent of pregnant women, is a darkening of the skin over the upper lip, cheeks, nose, and/or forehead. The pattern is blotchy and is caused by increased pigment deposits. The condition is more pronounced in dark-skinned women. It may appear anytime after the first trimester. Avoiding the sun and using sunscreen may help minimize the tone.

Q. *Will I have to live with this mask forever?*

A. Possibly. Melasma can be treated with prescription creams that will exfoliate or help remove the top layer of skin containing these pigments. If this treatment doesn't work, bleaching creams and steroid creams may be used. A chemical peel can be tried as well.

Q. *What other skin changes are common during pregnancy?*

A. There is also darkening of the areolas and nipples and a dark pigmented line extending from your pubic bone to your navel, called the *linea nigra*. It appears at the end of the first trimester. You may also notice the appearance of small freckles and moles. Spider veins (small red capillaries) may appear, most commonly on your chest. These blanch and fill when pressed, then fill back up with blood and are caused by the higher levels of estrogen. The appearance or disappearance of acne may be seen. These skin changes will not persist postpartum. If they do, your dermatologist can laser spider veins and remove skin tags.

Q. *Will I get stretch marks?*

A. I tell all my patients that they will get stretch marks, and I am correct 90 percent of the time. If your mom or sister had stretch marks, you will probably get these mommy marks as well. If you got stretch marks from gaining weight before, you will get more. If you got stretch marks during a previous pregnancy, you will get more in subsequent pregnancies. Stretch marks will most commonly occur to some degree on the abdomen, thighs, and breasts and can cause discomfort in the form of dryness and itching.

Q. *What can I do to prevent stretch marks?*

A. Nothing. Creams and oils will make your skin nice and soft but they will do nothing to prevent stretch marks.

Q. *Is it normal for my skin to be itchy during pregnancy?*

A. Yes, itching (pruritis) may occur to some degree in about 20 percent of pregnant women. A skin rash does not necessarily have to be present. The itching may occur over your entire body or be localized in one area, such as your abdomen. Itching is most intense at night and during hot, humid times of the year.

Q. *What can be done to relieve the itching?*

A. You can take baths with oatmeal soap and oil, use an antipruritic lotion containing menthol, or get a prescription for topical steroids and antihistamines from your doctor.

Q. *My palms and soles are red and itchy. What should I do?*

A. Avoid long hot showers and use fragrance-free soap, an OTC cold-mentholated lotion, or an oatmeal-based soap.

Q. *My skin feels very dry. What can I do?*

A. Use oil—any type from baby oil to walnut oil. It works.

Q. *Is there really a "glow of pregnancy"?*

A. Yes. All pregnant moms have an increase in blood volume and an increase in the blood flow to their skin. This will give you a redder complexion. The increase in tissue swelling will also temporarily decrease your fine lines and wrinkles.

Q. *Why does my belly button hurt?*

A. During pregnancy, your uterus expands and stretches the skin and muscles of your abdomen. There is a weak spot in your belly button that will stretch, too. The nerves in this area stretch, causing the discomfort.

Q. *My belly feels so heavy. What can I do?*

A. Try a maternity belt or girdle. There are many types. Find the one that works for you.

Q. *Why am I getting pimples on my face?*
And how can I get rid of them?

A. Your pregnancy hormones can cause the oil glands in your face to produce more oil, which can cause pimples. Wash your face morning and night with a good cleanser. Follow this with an astringent to remove the excess oil. Next apply an oil-free moisturizer.

Q. *These pimples are still out of control.*
What should I do?

A. After consulting with your doctor, you can use OTC benzoyl peroxide. For particularly severe cases of acne, topical clindamycin or erythromycin gel may be used. Never use Accutane (isotretinoin) if you are having unprotected sex or during your pregnancy. Topical Retin-A (tretinoin), also known as retinoic acid, is also contraindicated during pregnancy.

Q. *Is it normal to perspire a lot*
during pregnancy?

A. Yes, beginning in the third month of your pregnancy you will experience an increase in sweating due to an increase in thyroid gland secretion. This causes an increase in sweat, skin temperature, and redness. This excessive sweating commonly causes miliaria and intertrigo.

Q. *What is miliaria?*

A. Miliaria, also known as prickly heat or heat rash, is commonly experienced during pregnancy. The rash looks like tiny raised red bubbles and is itchy. Your discomfort may be eased by wearing loose clothing, reducing the humidity in your surroundings, and applying talcum powder or calamine lotion to affected areas. An oatmeal bath is both soothing and relaxing.

Q. *What is intertrigo?*

A. Intertrigo is a skin condition occurring in any skin area that is folded, such as the groin, underarms, abdomen, and under the breasts. The skin appears red and glazed and often becomes infected with *Candida albicans* (yeast) or bacteria. The skin area can burn or itch. Treatment consists of keeping these affected areas dry and clean. Hydrocortisone cream and an antifungal medication are sometimes required.

Q. *What are pruritic urticarial papules and plaques of pregnancy (PUPPP)?*

A. PUPPP is an intensely itchy (pruritic) skin eruption that occurs only during a pregnancy. The hives and red plaques first develop on the abdomen, usually around the navel, and then spread to the thighs and arms. The face is usually spared.

Q. *How common is PUPPP?*

A. PUPPP is the most common itchy skin disorder of pregnancy. It may occur in up to 1 percent of pregnancies. This skin disorder is more common in first pregnancies and seldom recurs in subsequent pregnancies. There are no adverse effects to your pregnancy from this dermatological disorder.

Q. *What is the treatment for PUPPP?*

A. The mainstay of treatment is topical corticosteroids. Antihistamines may also be tried for symptomatic relief of itching. Oral corticosteroids are used if the topicals do not work. The delivery of your baby is the ultimate cure; the rash and itching will fade within hours.

Q. *Why am I producing so much saliva?*
Is there a treatment?

A. There is an increased production of saliva by the salivary glands during pregnancy, which may infrequently be excessive (ptyalism). This annoying condition may cause nausea or may be caused by nausea or heartburn, may persist throughout pregnancy, and then disappears postpartum.

There is no specific treatment for excessive salivary gland output per se, but there are medicines you can try. An antihistamine may help, but the side effect of drowsiness that is common with antihistamines may be unbearable in an already fatigued state of pregnancy. However, drink a lot of fluids. You must replenish the fluids you are losing to prevent dehydration. If you have nausea or heartburn, treat it. Eat small meals frequently. Sweet (not sour) sucking candies will help you swallow the excess saliva.

Q. *Why do I feel swollen?*

A. Swelling normally occurs during the second and third trimesters. Remember, your body produces at least 6 quarts of fluid during your pregnancy. The extra fluid softens up the body so it can expand to accommodate your growing baby and soften your joints so you can expand to deliver your baby. This swelling is called *edema* and is actually excess water in these tissues. It occurs most commonly in the third trimester owing to the weight of the uterus pressing on the main veins. This pressure slows down the return of blood from your legs and allows the water in the vessels to move out into the surrounding tissue in your legs, most notably in your ankles and feet. Swelling is particularly problematic during hot weather.

Q. *How can I prevent or relieve this swelling?*

A. To relieve swelling:

- Try not to stand in place for long periods at a time. Move your feet and calves around; this helps pump the blood out of your legs.
- Restrict your intake of salty foods.
- Don't wear tight half-length nylons.
- If you are able to, keep your toes above your nose when sitting or lying down.

Q. *I have a vaginal discharge. Is it an infection?*

A. If the discharge burns, itches, has a bad odor, or makes your vulva red and swollen, you may have an infection. If you have none of these complaints, you have the normal increased vaginal secretions that occur during pregnancy. This discharge may be clear or white and becomes mucoid near term.

Q. *Why did I get red marks on my face and chest? Will I always have them?*

A. These are called spider veins and are tiny blood vessels growing in the surface of your skin. These spider veins usually disappear postpartum. If they don't, laser treatment is effective in eradicating them.

Q. *When am I likely to develop varicose veins?*

A. Varicose veins commonly occur near the end of the second trimester. They are due to the pressure of the pregnant uterus on the main veins, slowing down the blood flow and distending the veins in the legs and/or vulva. The veins are easily distended because their tone is already decreased by the effects of progesterone. Varicose veins tend to occur in families; ask your mother if she has them.

Q. *What is the treatment for varicose veins during pregnancy?*

A. Treatment during pregnancy is for the symptomatic relief of pain only and usually includes the following:

- Try maternity support hose first. If this does not relieve your symptoms, you may be fitted with elastic stockings by your doctor.
- A pregnancy girdle will relieve tension in vulvar varicosities.
- When possible, keep your toes above your nose.
- Don't stand in one place for long periods of time.

Q. *Are vulvar varicosities common?*

A. Yes, and they are more common with each pregnancy and with advanced age. They are not dangerous. Occasionally, the varicose vein could bleed and you could confuse it with vaginal bleeding. Check to see where the bleeding is coming from. A clot in a varicose vein in your leg is not dangerous, but it can give you a dull throbbing pain. A superficial vein thrombosis cannot release a clot that can travel to your brain, heart, or lungs. Only a deep vein throbosis (DVT) potentially can.

CHAPTER 4

Diet and Nutrition

Q. *Why do I have to gain weight during my pregnancy?*

A. Pregnancy causes certain organs of the body to grow to support the developing fetus. Remember, your baby also adds weight to your body. Studies have shown that the best outcome of a pregnancy—a healthy baby—occurs when the mother gains an adequate amount of weight.

Q. *Does my prepregnancy weight have any effect on my baby's weight?*

A. Yes, thin women tend to have smaller babies than women whose weight is in the normal range for the same given weight gain during pregnancy. Overweight women tend to have heavier babies independent of their gestational weight gain.

Q. *My prepregnancy weight was in the normal range. How much weight should I gain?*

A. You should gain at least 24 pounds and no more than 35 pounds. This is easily achieved by a diet supplying 2,400 calories per day. For all prepregnancy weights, the average weight gain has been recorded at about 33 pounds in some studies. Don't be overly concerned with weight gain; you will gain weight. Place your emphasis on eating the proper foods.

Q. *I was underweight before I became*
     pregnant. How much weight should I gain?

A. Underweight women should gain at least 30 to 35 pounds. Your increased weight gain will have a greater influence on the weight gain of your baby, bringing his or her weight into the normal range.

Q. *I was very overweight before I became*
     pregnant. How much weight should I gain?

A. There is no minimal weight gain for the overweight pregnant woman. However, you should be concerned with the quality of your diet. For you, proper nutrition and exercise as supervised by your doctor will ensure good growth for your baby. Inadequate nutrition will have an effect on the development of your baby, so don't diet.

Q. *If my prepregnancy weight is not in*
     the normal range, am I at an
     increased risk for miscarriage?

A. There is no relationship between prepregnancy weight and miscarriages.

Q. *How many extra calories do*
     I need daily during my pregnancy?

A. The Food and Nutrition Board recommends an extra 300 calories per day (300 calories is equal to 2½ cups of low-fat milk,

a cup of ice cream, a bagel with cream cheese, or a turkey sand-
wich). To maintain her weight before becoming pregnant, the average woman requires 2,000 calories per day. The 300 additional
calories are an average throughout your pregnancy. Don't be worried if you are nauseous in the beginning of your pregnancy and
can't eat. The need for additional calories is greater in the last
trimester, when you may consume a total caloric intake of 2,500 or
more calories per day.

Q. *Do I have to gain any fat
during my pregnancy?*

A. You do not have to put on a large amount of weight in the
form of fat, but a small amount of weight gain that is fat may help
in the growth of the fetus.

Q. *How much weight should I gain
throughout the trimesters?*

A. The typical weight gain in the first trimester is 3 to 8 pounds.
It is usually not a problem if you do not gain any weight; however,
a large weight gain by underweight women is usually desirable. In
the second trimester, a weight gain of 10 to 15 pounds is desired. It
has been shown that a smaller weight gain during this time is corre-
lated with an increased risk of delivering an IUGR (intrauterine
growth retardation) baby. During your third trimester, the recommended weight gain is 10 to 15 pounds. Some of this weight gain
may be due to edema in your legs. This is okay because we know that
this type of edema is associated with improved fetal growth.

Q. *How can I gain the weight?*

A. Gaining weight during pregnancy is easy. Putting the weight on properly is the hard part; a fast-food diet is not the way. Now that you are pregnant, it is time to prepare for parenthood by nourishing your baby properly. A well-rounded diet from the four basic food groups is the key to proper nutrition, caloric intake, and weight gain during pregnancy. If you eat the proper foods, according to your appetite, you will achieve these goals.

Q. *What are the risks of not gaining enough or gaining too much weight during my pregnancy?*

A. With inadequate weight gain, you risk delivering your baby prematurely. There is also a risk of about 15 percent of having an underweight or growth-restricted baby.

Women who begin their pregnancy at or above the normal prepregnancy weight and who gain more than the recommended amount of weight during their pregnancy may deliver babies who will weigh more. This may increase your chances of having a dysfunctional labor, vacuum or forceps delivery, shoulder dystocia (the head is delivered easily but there is difficulty delivering the baby's shoulders), clavicular (collarbone) fracture (of the baby), and cesarean section. However, a greater-than-normal weight gain will not cause your baby to weigh a lot more. For each additional 10 pounds of weight gain, the average increase in your baby's birth weight will be about 3 ounces. Gaining a large amount of weight will contribute to your overall discomfort: an increased probability of back, hip, and leg pain and an increased risk of developing varicose veins.

Of course, pregnancy in general, and pregnancy weight gain in particular, is associated with retained maternal weight in the postpartum period. If you gain the recommended 30 pounds during your pregnancy, you will lose about 26 pounds in the early postpartum period. If you gain 50 pounds during your pregnancy, you will still lose only 26 pounds in the early postpartum period.

Q. *I'm gaining too much weight but I'm really not eating that much. What's going on?*

A. I've heard that before. But really you are eating too much—or the small amount of food that you are eating is packed with a lot of calories. Fast foods are packed with fat calories, so even though the portions are relatively small, the the number of weight-inducing calories are not. The same goes with beverages. Check the calories on the fluids you are drinking. For example, if you started drinking two glasses of whole milk each day, that would add an extra 320 calories per day to your intake. That satisfies the increased daily recommended requirement of calories needed during pregnancy. The problem is, it does not satisfy your daily appetite requirement. So you unknowingly eat your extra 300 calories per day as well and don't understand the increased weight gain.

Q. *I am hungry all the time, I am eating all the time, and I am gaining more than 1 pound per week. What can I do?*

A. Some women develop a voracious appetite and a bottomless pit for a stomach. The first line of strategy is to make better food choices. For example, instead of snacking on potato or tortilla chips, eat cleaned raw vegetables, either plain or with a low-calorie dressing or salsa. Pickles are another good snack food. They are low in calories and there are an assortment of types—dill, bread and butter, half sour, sour, and sweet. Fruit is another healthy snack food. Remember to drink low-calorie fluids constantly throughout the day; this will fill your belly and help curb you appetite. Before you eat your meal, have either a salad with low-calorie dressing, such as balsamic or rice vinegar, or a bowl of chicken broth, or both. That should let you enjoy a smaller portion of dinner and save you some calories.

Q. *Does my gestational weight gain have an effect on my ability to breast-feed?*

A. No. Your weight gain during pregnancy has little impact on the quantity or quality of your breast milk.

NUTRITION

Q. *Who is at high risk for a nutritional problem?*

A. Those at high risk include:

- Under- and overweight women
- Early-teenage women
- Women with a multiple pregnancy (twins or triplets)
- Anemic women
- Anorexics or bulimics
- Drug and/or alcohol abusers
- Heavy cigarette smokers
- Strict vegetarians
- Women who maintain a high level of physical activity

Q. *If I am in a high-risk category,*
what should I do?

A. If you are in one or more of the high-risk categories, an increased supply of selected nutrients may be indicated. This is most easily accomplished with food because an increased need for certain minerals and vitamins is also accompanied by an increased need for energy and for other nutrients that are not provided by a multivitamin-mineral product.

Q. *What types of foods are in the*
protein group?

A. Beans, eggs, fish, meat, nuts, peas, poultry and seeds. Choose meats and poultry that are lean and lower in fat. Nuts, seeds, and fish are packed with healthy oils and should be a larger part of your diet from this group. Foods from the protein group supply you and your baby with protein, B vitamins, and iron. These nutrients are used to build and maintain bone, muscle, blood cells, skin, and nerves. B vitamins are needed for energy, for building red blood cells and other tissues, and for proper functioning of your nervous system. Iron is needed in your red blood cells to carry oxygen.

Q. *Do I need extra calcium in my diet?*

A. Calcium is necessary for the formation of bones in your baby's skeleton. Your growing baby requires calcium during its development. If you do not supply calcium through your diet, you will supply the calcium from your own stores—your bones. This could potentially lead to osteoporosis (demineralization of the bone). It is recommended that pregnant women increase their calcium intake by an extra 600 milligrams for a total of about 1,500 milligrams a day. If you take a supplement, take one that provides 600 milligrams of elemental calcium per day. It is a good idea to take your calcium tablet at the end of a light meal to promote absorption of the calcium.

Q. *What are good food sources of calcium?*

A. The best sources are milk, cheese, and yogurt. One glass of milk contains 300 milligrams of calcium. In addition, many foods and drinks are now fortified with calcium.

Q. *I have lactose intolerance.*
What should I do?

A. You may be able to tolerate small amounts of milk, for example, ½ cup at a time. Whole milk may be better tolerated than skim or nonfat milk. You may be able to tolerate yogurt, hard cheeses, or low-lactose milk. Try lactase tablets, which help digest lactose. In addition, here are good sources of calcium equal to 1 cup of milk:

- 3 ounces of sardines if the bones are eaten
- 6 ounces of canned salmon if the bones are eaten
- 8 ounces of tofu if processed with calcium sulfate
- Two waffles or four pancakes
- 9 ounces of shrimp
- Other foods containing calcium, such as collards, bok choy, turnip greens, kale, broccoli, and cooked oysters

Q. *Why should I eat foods from the fruit and vegetable groups?*

A. These foods provide you and your baby with vitamins A, C, and E, fiber, and potassium. Vitamin A is needed to resist infections, and it also keeps your skin healthy and your eyes sharp, especially at night. Vitamin C is needed for good wound healing and for maintaining healthy teeth and gums. Vitamin E prevents essential fatty acids and vitamin A from being destroyed. Dietary fiber reduces your blood cholesterol level, maintains good bowel function, and is a low-calorie filling food. Potassium is needed to maintain normal blood pressure, reduce the risk of forming kidney stones, and prevent bone loss. A diet high in fruits and vegetables will also reduce the risk of stroke; mouth, stomach, and colon cancer; and the development of type 2 diabetes.

Q. *Which foods make up the grain group?*

A. Barley, bran, cornmeal, oats, rice, and wheat. Grains are either whole grains or refined grains. Whole grains contain the entire kernel, such as brown rice, whole wheat, and (my favorite) popcorn. Refined grains do not include the bran and germ; examples are white flour and white rice. Foods whose labels start with "brown rice," "bulgur," "graham flour," "oatmeal," "whole-grain corn," "whole oats," "whole rye," "whole wheat," or "wild rice" are whole-grain foods. Foods whose labels list "bran," "cracked wheat," "multigrain," "seven-grain," "stone-ground," or "100% wheat" are not whole-grain foods.

Other foods, such as pastries, fats, and spices, do make eating more enjoyable. They will provide you with some extra calories that you may or may not need, as the case may be. Limit your diet to a minimum of foods containing empty calories. Eat yogurt, ice milk, or puddings instead of chips or candy.

Q. *Which foods contain protein?*

A. Protein is necessary for the growth, development, and maintenance of your tissues and those of the fetus. Protein is made up of smaller units called amino acids. There are twenty different amino acids. Your body can produce twelve of them. The other eight are called the "essential" amino acids and must be eaten because your body cannot manufacture them.

Protein is found in red meats, poultry, fish, and dairy products. These are complete protein foods, meaning they contain all the essential amino acids and can be eaten alone for an adequate source of protein. Many vegetables also contain protein, but each vegetable lacks one or more of the eight essential amino acids. If you are a vegetarian, you must learn to combine your protein sources to take in all the essential amino acids. The recommended amount of protein is about 60 to 80 grams per day, depending on your weight.

Q. *Can I drink a high-protein beverage or amino acid supplement during my pregnancy?*

A. Although there is no question of the benefits of adequate protein intake during pregnancy, excessive protein intake may be harmful. Several studies have shown that the addition of specially formulated high-protein supplements has led to an increase in preterm labor and a decrease in birth weight.

Q. *What are omega-3 fatty acids?*

A. These are fatty acids found in dark fish and certain nuts. The most important omega-3 fatty acid is docosahexaenoic acid (DHA). The level of DHA in your blood decreases during pregnancy.

Q. *Why should I take an omega-3 fatty acid supplement?*

A. Omega-3 fatty acid is needed for proper brain and eye development in the fetus. In fact, 40 percent of the fat in your baby's developing brain and eyes comes from omega-3 fatty acid. Supplemental omega-3 fatty acid will also decrease your risk of preterm labor, especially if you have a past history of preterm labor.

Q. *Which foods contain iron?*

A. There are two types of food that contain iron: animal products, which contain heme iron (iron derived from hemoglobin, which is found in blood), and plant products, which contain nonheme iron. Most of your dietary iron will be supplied through plant products, such as apricots, beans, nuts, pumpkin seeds, and spinach. A fortified breakfast cereal cannot prevent anemia during pregnancy. Breakfast cereals in the United States typically are not fortified with ferrous iron. Those cereals that do contain iron are also rich in phytates, which inhibit the absorption of nonheme iron.

Q. *Do I need extra folic acid during pregnancy?*

A. Yes. Extra folic acid is needed for the production of red blood cells in both the mother and the fetus. In addition, according to the

U.S. Public Health Service, any woman who is even capable of be-coming pregnant should take a vitamin that contains 0.4 milligram of folic acid to reduce the incidence of neural tube defects such as spina bifida or anencephaly in the fetus.

Folates are found in high amounts in leafy green vegetables, asparagus, broccoli, avocados, okra, brussel sprouts, and corn. Folic acid is also found in many fortified foods, such as breads and cereals and, of course, in your prenatal vitamin.

Q. *How much fluid should I drink each day?*

A. You should drink about eight to ten glasses of fluids a day. Milk, fruit juices, soups, and water all count as liquids. So do carbonated beverages, but they are either diet (contain aspartame or saccharin) or nondiet (contain quite a number of calories). Sodas, fruit juices with added fructose, and alcohol are liquids that should be avoided.

Q. *Should I limit my intake of salt (sodium)?*

A. No. You may salt your foods to taste. There is no reason to re-strict your salt intake. Salt is not the cause of toxemia, as was once believed. In fact, during pregnancy, the requirement for sodium is increased. Of course, if you are experiencing annoying swelling of your ankles and feet, you may want to restrict your salt intake somewhat. Foods that contain a high salt content are canned, pack-aged, or frozen foods, fast foods, cold cuts, and pickles.

Q. *How much fat should my diet contain?*

A. Fats provide energy and are necessary for the absorption of the fat-soluble vitamins D, E, A, and K, and calcium. There is an essential fat called linoleic acid that is not produced by your body but that is necessary for the growth and maintenance of your tissues. Try to limit your fat intake to between 20 and (at most) 35 percent of your diet. Try to consume fats that are composed of monounsaturated or polyunsaturated fatty acids. The best sources of these types of fatty acids are fish, nuts, and vegetable oils. You will want to try to limit the amount of fats and oils that are high in saturated or trans-fatty acids, which are found in solid fats.

Examples of solid fats are butter or stick margarine, many cheeses and creams, bakery items such as cookies and doughnuts, and bacon, sausages, poultry skin, marbled beef, and regular ground beef (fast-food hamburgers). Animal meats and products that contain solid fats also contain cholesterol. Vegetable oils do not contain cholesterol. The only common vegetable oil to avoid is coconut oil, which is high in saturated fats and is used to make theater popcorn. If you follow the diet guidelines I have given for eating animal proteins and grains, you will obtain a sufficient amount of fat.

Q. *How much carbohydrate should my diet contain?*

A. Carbohydrates contain B vitamins and vitamin C and are also a quick source of energy. There are some forms of carbohydrates that are not nutritious, however. These are the refined sugars (white or brown sugar, honey, or molasses). They are quick sources of energy, calories, and weight gain. Try to eat foods containing complex carbohydrates instead, such as fruits, vegetables, grains, and cereals. These foods also contain a healthy amount of fiber, which will prevent constipation.

Q. *Do pregnant women really have cravings for certain foods?*

A. Yes. Sometimes a woman may crave citrus fruits because she actually needs more vitamin C or a sweet because she has hypoglycemia (low blood sugar) at that time, usually in the middle of the night. Other food cravings may be more unusual—for instance, the practice of eating laundry starch, clay, or ice shavings from a freezer. This is called pica and may be due to severe iron deficiency, although this is not always the case. Still, it is a common practice among pregnant women in impoverished areas. It is estimated that between 75 and 90 percent of pregnant women crave at least one food item.

Q. *Do some pregnant women have aversions to certain foods?*

A. Yes. You may even develop a dislike for foods that you usually enjoy. Between 50and 85 percent of women report aversions to at least one type of food during pregnancy.

Q. *Is it safe for me to use aspartame (NutraSweet) during my pregnancy?*

A. Aspartame is made from two amino acids, aspartic acid and phenylalanine, which are building blocks for protein. The Food and Drug Administration (FDA) has approved the use of aspartame as a safe food ingredient for pregnant women. The American Academy of

Pediatrics Committee on Nutrition has also approved aspartame as safe to use during pregnancy for both the mother and the developing fetus. Only women with PKU (phenylketonuria), a rare chemical birth defect that prevents them from oxidizing phenylalanine, should restrict their use of artificial sweeteners, as the resulting accumulation of phenylalanine may cause mental retardation in the fetus.

Q. *Can I use saccharin during my pregnancy?*

A. Saccharin may be used during pregnancy. It is not digested and passes through your intestines unchanged. Saccharin does cross the placenta, but there is no evidence that it is harmful to your fetus. Still, saccharin has been linked to bladder cancer if used in high amounts in adults, so why start your baby off early? Avoid it.

Q. *Can I use Splenda during pregnancy?*

A. Yes. Splenda is sucralose, made from sugar and another noncalorie sweetener. The FDA has approved Splenda for consumption during pregnancy. Low-calorie sweeteners can be useful to pregnant women who have diabetes, who need to control their calorie intake, or who enjoy the taste of these sweeteners. Women without health or weight problems should not use sugar substitutes to restrict calorie intake. Remember, calorie intake should increase during pregnancy.

Q. *Can I eat foods made with sugar alcohol?*

A. Yes. Sugar alcohols are isomalt mannitol, sorbitol, and xylitol. They are found in many dietetic foods labeled as sugar free or low carb. These foods can be consumed in moderation during pregnancy.

Q. *Can I eat foods that contain Sunett?*

A. Yes. Sunett, or acesulfane potassium, is found in dietetic foods and is FDA safe during pregnancy.

Q. *Is it safe to eat foods that are labeled "low fat" or "fat free"?*

A. Yes. Most low-fat foods use carbohydrates in place of fat. There are different types of carbohydrates used, such as cornstarch, oat bran, and even seaweed. Fat-free foods may contain the fat-substitute protein compound Simplesse.

FISH

Q. *Can I eat fish when I am pregnant?*

A. Yes. Fish is an excellent source of lean protein, low in saturated fats and high in omega-3 fatty acids. You may eat 12 ounces of fish per week, which is equal to two meals a week. If you don't eat any fish during a given week, you may eat more than two meals of fish during the next week. However, fish contains traces of methylmercury, which in large doses can be harmful to your fetus. Methylmercury is the compound that forms when mercury mixes with water. Fish slowly accumulate methylmercury in their tissues throughout their lives. A regular diet of fish with a high content of methylmercury during pregnancy will expose your fetus to this chemical. High doses of methylmercury can damage your baby's developing nervous system, causing learning disabilities and other developmental delays.

Q. *Which fish are safe to eat?*

A. It's safe to eat wild salmon, chunk light canned tuna, sardines, shrimp, blue crab, farmed trout and catfish, fish sticks, fast-food fish sandwiches, summer flounder, haddock, and pollock. If you are craving it, you can eat tuna, but 6 ounces of albacore tuna should be counted as your two meals of the week.

Q. *Which fish should I absolutely avoid eating?*

A. Avoid large fish, including king mackerel, shark, swordfish, and tilefish as advised by the FDA. Other fish that should be omitted from your diet are tuna steak, halibut, marlin, sea bass, and pike.

Q. *Can I eat raw fish sushi during my pregnancy?*

A. No. Most fish used in preparing sushi are from the large-fish variety containing a higher concentration of methylmercury. You should also avoid eating raw oysters during your pregnancy.

Q. *Can I eat fish caught by myself or by my family or friends?*

A. The answer depends on the level of methylmercury in the waters the fish came from. You can check the local fish advisories for this information or go to the website epa.gov/ost/fish.

Q. *Can I eat deli meats when I am pregnant?*

A. Yes. Just reheat the meat until the meat is steaming. This will protect you from an infection with listeria.

Q. *What is listeria?*

A. *Listeria monocytogenes* is a bacterium that is commonly found in water. It can be found in uncooked foods, imported cheeses, and deli meats. Listeria can infect your bloodstream and pass through the placenta and infect the placenta and your fetus. This infection could cause a miscarriage, premature delivery, and infection to the baby. Fortunately, listeria infections are not very common during pregnancy. Each year about 675 pregnant women will become infected.

With listeria, you will have mild flu-like symptoms, which can appear up to 30 days after exposure. Severe infections, if they occur, are usually during the third trimester, when the immune system is the most suppressed. Severe infections are characterized by high fever, severe abdominal pain, and labor pains. The infection can be treated with antibiotics, which will prevent infection in your baby.

Q. *Can I eat soft cheeses during my pregnancy?*

A. Yes, if they are made in the United States with pasteurized milk. Imported soft cheeses should not be eaten. These cheeses include Brie, Camembert, feta, Gorgonzola, queso blanco, queso fresco, and Roquefort. These cheeses may contain listeria.

Q. *Can I eat pâté?*

A. No. Pâté may be contaminated with listeria.

Q. *I am a lacto-ovovegetarian.*
Should I alter my diet when I am pregnant?

A. No, but you should supplement your diet with 30 milligrams of elemental iron a day and 15 milligrams of zinc, which are found in most prenatal vitamins.

Q. *I am a vegan. Should I change my diet?*

A. You must combine your foods to provide for all the amino acids needed to form the proteins your baby requires to grow. Since most vegetables do not contain large amounts of the essential amino acids (amino acids that your body cannot synthesize), expect to eat an abundant amount of food every day and therefore expect to gain much more than 30 pounds during your pregnancy.

VITAMINS AND SUPPLEMENTS

Q. *Which prenatal vitamin should I take?*

A. If you eat three well-balanced meals a day, you will meet the requirements for vitamins and minerals required each day and will not need a vitamin supplement. Unfortunately, many pregnant women, for a variety of reasons (morning sickness, food cravings or aversions, "too busy"), do not eat properly and may benefit from taking a prenatal vitamin. Prenatal vitamins are supplements and should not be used as a substitute for food. Each doctor has his or her own preference of prescription or over-the-counter (OTC) brands. Just remember to take your pill with food for better absorption. If you can't swallow pills, ask your doctor about taking children's chewable vitamins.

Q. *My doctor said that I was anemic and advised me to start taking an iron pill in addition to my prenatal vitamin. What kinds of iron preparations are available?*

A. There are three types of iron supplement preparations to choose from: plain iron, slow-release iron, and iron with ascorbic acid (vitamin C). In addition, each of these preparations can contain three different types of iron compounds: ferrous sulfate, ferrous gluconate, and ferrous fumarate.

Q. *Which iron preparation should I use?*

A. Each of the preparations has its advantages and disadvantages. Plain iron is the least expensive, but because it must be taken between meals on an empty stomach, it may cause heartburn, nausea, and upper abdominal discomfort. Slow-release preparations decrease these side effects and may be taken with meals, although maximal absorption still occurs if taken in between meals. Iron with ascorbic acid may enhance the absorption of iron, but it is more expensive than plain iron—and the ascorbic acid may cause additional upper abdominal discomfort. Taking this preparation with a meal is not recommended.

Q. *Before I became pregnant, I took megavitamins. Can I continue to do so during my pregnancy?*

A. The use of megavitamins can be dangerous, whether you are pregnant or not. High doses of vitamin B_6 for prolonged periods of time may cause neurological problems, such as numbness or tingling in your hands and feet. Vitamin A toxicity can cause fatigue, brittle nails, hair loss, scaly skin, joint pain, and abdominal pain. Your baby may be born with increased pressure in the spinal column and brain, bone decalcification, growth retardation, or possible abnormalities of the urinary tract system.

High doses of vitamin D for prolonged periods may cause nausea, vomiting, anorexia, hypertension, and calcium deposits in tissues other than your bones. Your baby could be born with mental retardation or a cleft palate. Megadoses of vitamin C may cause kidney stones in you and scurvy in your baby because the increased amount in the womb makes the infant require more vitamin C.

CHAPTER 5

Health and Fitness Concerns

Q. *Do stress and anxiety affect the fetus?*

A. Yes and no. It is very common for pregnant women to experience mood swings throughout the day and throughout their pregnancy. You may at times become intensely angry or depressed and suffer from crying spells. Studies have found that if there is an increased risk of miscarriage from stress, the risk is extremely small and may be attributed to the way the stress is dealt with, such as cigarette smoking or drug or alcohol abuse. Medical research has shown that the everyday stress and anxiety of life in no way affect the health and well-being of your fetus. However, there is evidence that acute stress can cause miscarriages, birth defects, or preterm labor.

If you are concerned about the increased level of stress in your life, talk to your doctor. Of course, high levels of stress for long periods of time can affect your health whether you are pregnant or not. You may experience high blood pressure, or your resistance to infections may be lowered. And if you have diabetes, stress can make your blood sugar hard to control. During pregnancy, you may also experience a slightly increased risk of preeclampsia. You may have a low-birth-weight baby as a result of poor coping habits due to a lack of appetite and inadequate caloric intake.

Q. *What should I know about bathing during pregnancy?*

A. In general, baths during pregnancy are safe as long as you take a few precautions. Do not bathe in water so hot that it could raise your core body temperature. You will know when your core body temperature is elevated because you will become uncomfortably warm. This is pretty hard to do, since the bath water cools fairly quickly. The greatest risk to the fetus is during the first 6 weeks of your pregnancy, during the formation of the spinal cord. A high core temperature could cause a neural tube defect in your fetus, causing spina bifida.

If you know you are pregnant, just take warm baths during early pregnancy. If you need to wash in hot water, take a hot shower. Hot showers cannot raise your core body temperature. Near the end of the second trimester and throughout the third trimester, make sure someone is home with you when you bathe. Remember, your center of balance has changed owing to your enlarging uterus, which makes slipping and falling an easy thing to do. Do not take a bath if your membranes have ruptured and you are leaking amniotic fluid; instead, take a shower before going to the hospital. A nice warm bath may help those of you who are having trouble falling asleep at night.

Q. *I was in a hot tub last week before I realized that I was pregnant. Did I harm my baby?*

A. Some studies have shown an increased risk of miscarriage and neural tube defects in women who had high fevers during the first 6 weeks of pregnancy. For this reason, we recommend not using a hot tub for extended times during early pregnancy. The danger potentially occurs when the core body temperature reaches 102°F. This takes about 20 minutes if your hot tub is set at 104°F. Most people cannot stay in a hot tub for that long, so don't get hot and bothered.

Q. *Then can I use a hot tub during the rest of my pregnancy?*

A. Sure, as long as the temperature of the water is equal to your body temperature. The same potential infections may occur from contaminated water as in a pool (see page 98). In addition, a bacterial infection called *pseudomonas* may be contracted, causing a skin rash.

Q. *Can I sunbathe during my pregnancy?*

A. Yes, sunbathing is not harmful to your pregnancy, but it is probably not the best choice for your skin. Tanning will cause your skin to wrinkle earlier in life and it increases your risk for some skin cancers. If you still want to sunbathe, use a suntan lotion that contains SPF (sun protection factor) 30 or more. Stay cool and drink plenty of fluids to prevent raising your core body temperature and to avoid dehydration. However, if you are prone to developing chloasma, this will intensify your mask of pregnancy, so avoid the sun or at least wear a hat.

Q. *Can I go to a tanning salon?*

A. Yes, but the same precautions apply as in the previous answer. In addition, remember that if you get dizzy or nauseous lying on your back, you will not be able to tolerate a tanning bed.

Q. *Can I use sunless tanning products while pregnant?*

A. Most definitely. This is the best way to get a tan before, during, and after your pregnancy. These products are safe to use during pregnancy, and the products are becoming better and better at simulating a natural tan without harming your skin with UV rays.

Q. *Can I get a new pair of contact lenses during my pregnancy?*

A. It's not advisable. There are temporary changes in the cornea of your eye, which can change your eyesight. There is also a change in the composition of your tears that may cause your contact lenses to become greasy. Discomfort is caused by swelling of the cornea. This is most common near the end of pregnancy.

Q. *Can I douche when I am pregnant?*

A. I do not recommend routine douching, whether you are pregnant or not. However, some women cannot stand the excessive vaginal discharge occasionally present during pregnancy. If you must douche, do not use a bulb syringe; deaths to pregnant women from an air embolism have occurred. To prevent high pressure, the douche bag should not be placed more than 2 feet above your hips, and do not insert the nozzle more than 3 inches into your vagina. You will discover that if you have a normal vaginal discharge called leukorrhea during pregnancy, the douche you just performed was worthless because you will notice the same amount of vaginal discharge within a few hours.

Q. *Should I go to the dentist when
I am pregnant?*

A. Your routine dental checkups should continue when you are
pregnant. If this was a planned pregnancy, hopefully you have had
your checkup already. If you have dental caries or need any procedures done, try waiting until the second trimester.

Q. *Should I have dental X-rays taken
during pregnancy?*

A. If your dentist feels you need X-rays, have them done. The
X-rays are directed away from your abdomen, which is shielded with
a lead apron. There is little danger to your developing fetus. Still,
always try to schedule your dental X-rays in the second trimester.

Q. *If I need dental work done, what kind
of anesthesia is safe for my dentist to use?*

A. The safest form of anesthesia for the pregnant patient is local anesthesia. Nitrous oxide, general anesthesia, and intravenous
sedatives should be avoided.

Q. *Can I get my teeth cleaned
during pregnancy?*

A. Can you? Yes. Should you? Most definitely. Pregnancy hormones will make your gums swell, and more food particles than
usual will get trapped in between your teeth and gums. Regular
professional teeth cleaning will prevent periodontal (gum) disease.

Q. *I have periodontitis. Should I wait until
I am postpartum to get a deep cleaning?*

A. No. Recent studies have revealed that periodontal disease may increase the incidence of preterm labor. Treatment of periodontal disease during pregnancy will reduce this risk of preterm labor. Another study showed an increased risk of preeclampsia in women who had periodontal disease. Now you have another reason to keep those gums healthy with regular brushing, flossing, and dental appointments.

Q. *My dentist wants me to take
antibiotics. Is that okay?*

A. If you are not allergic to the antibiotic, you may take penicillin, amoxicillin, cephalosporin, or clindamycin.

Q. *Do I need a fluoride supplement
during pregnancy?*

A. Adults in general may derive some benefit in the prevention of dental caries by drinking fluorinated water. However, fluoride supplementation during pregnancy has not been endorsed by the American Dental Association. In fact, mottled enamel (dental fluorosis) has occurred in developing teeth in areas where there is too much fluoride in the water supply.

Q. *Can I have a permanent when I am pregnant?*

A. Permanents are safe during pregnancy; however, some women experience thinning of their hair and may want to wait until after delivery for a new hairstyle.

Q. *Can I get my hair straightened*
during my pregnancy?

A. Yes. No birth defects or obstetrical complications have been reported.

Q. *Can I dye my hair during pregnancy?*

A. Although there are no known developmental risks to your baby, it is advised that you dye your hair after the first trimester. But if you unknowingly dyed your hair in the first trimester, don't worry. There is no evidence that hair dyes cause any harm to your baby.

Q. *Can I wear acrylic nails and nail*
polish during my pregnancy?

A. Yes. Acrylic nails and nail polishes contain solvents that have been found to be safe to use during pregnancy. Of course, it is a good idea to apply these cosmetics in a well-ventilated area.

Q. *Can I get a bikini or Brazilian wax*
during my pregnancy?

A. Sure, as often as you want to.

Q. *What kind of bra should I buy during pregnancy?*

A. Cotton maternity bras offer the best support for your enlarging breasts. It is possible for you to change two or three cup sizes during your pregnancy. If your breasts are pendulous, you may want to wear a bra all the time. Buy your nursing bra a few weeks before your due date, and make sure it is one size larger than the bra you are wearing at the time.

Q. *When should I take off my rings?*

A. Not every pregnant woman has to remove her rings, but if a ring is starting to feel tight on your finger, take it off. If you wait too long, you will have to have it removed by the jeweler. A tight-fitting ring can act like a tourniquet and stop the blood flow to your finger. If you are embarrassed to be seen pregnant and without your wedding ring, have your loved one buy a necklace to put your ring on!

Q. *I have a belly button ring, nipple rings, and a genital ring. Do I have to remove any or all of them during my pregnancy?*

A. No. There is no increased risk of infection if you had these piercings before you became pregnant. However, if the piercings do become uncomfortable because of your increased weight gain and swelling, you should remove them. You can replace the stud or ring with clean fishing line yourself or go to your piercing parlor and have them replace your studs with their own flexible jewelry. If you have decided that you will not replace your piercing after your pregnancy, take the rings out early to prevent unsightly scarring.

Q. *Can I get body piercing during my pregnancy?*

A. It is not recommended because the holes don't heal well as you body is growing and the site is more prone to infection during pregnancy.

Q. *I got a new tattoo last week and just found out that I am pregnant. Did I harm my baby?*

A. There is no information about the safety of skin dyes used in tattoos during pregnancy. I suspect that the risk to the fetus is negligible if risky at all. There is a slightly increased risk of skin infections during pregnancy as a result of your weakened immune system, so I would wait. Also, where are you going to put your tattoo? Anyplace on your body is going to grow and swell. The tattoo can become distorted during and after your pregnancy, when you are back down to your normal weight.

Q. *I have a tattoo across my lower back. Can I still get an epidural or spinal?*

A. The anesthesiologist will administer an epidural or spinal even if you have a tattoo in the area the needle will enter.

Q. *Can I cook with a microwave oven during my pregnancy?*

A. It is safe to cook with a microwave oven during pregnancy. The microwaves are shielded by several safety features built into the oven. There is a possibility that you could be exposed to some microwaves from a leak in the door, but you would have to stand directly in front of the oven for several hours to receive any significant exposure. The energy of the waves becomes progressively weaker the farther you are from the oven, so even a leaking microwave could be used without any adverse consequences.

Q. *Can I sleep with an electric blanket during my pregnancy?*

A. There are some studies showing an increased rate of miscarriage in women who sleep under electric blankets during pregnancy, and there are other studies that show no increased risks. The use of an electric blanket will not increase your core body temperature enough to cause a neural tube defect. In any case, use a warm body or quilt to keep you warm during those winter months.

Q. *Can I paint my baby's room if I am pregnant?*

A. Yes, if you must. There is probably very little risk to your baby from using paints that are acrylic, enamel, latex, or even oil based. It would still be wiser to have someone else do the painting. If you have to paint the nursery, keep the room well ventilated and take frequent breaks to limit your exposure to the fumes. If you are in your third trimester, avoid painting on a ladder; your balance is not the best. If you painted a room before you discovered that you were pregnant, have no fear; there is no evidence that household paints cause birth defects or miscarriage.

Q. *Can I use household cleaning products when I am pregnant?*

A. Unfortunately, you can. Studies have shown that household exposure to these agents has not caused an increase in birth defects or pregnancy complications. When using any chemical, remember to ventilate the area well. The use of rubber gloves is another good precaution.

Q. *Does loud noise affect the fetus?*

A. Yes it does, but not adversely. A loud noise such as you would experience at a rock concert or at an airport is also heard by your fetus. The noise evokes a startle response in both you and your baby. The baby will react by moving and by experiencing an increased heart rate. This is a very healthy response to the noise. In fact, medical research is currently being done using sound to evoke this reaction and correlating it with fetal well-being.

Q. *Can I use pesticides in the house*
   when I am pregnant?

A. You may have your dwelling sprayed with insecticides, just don't do it yourself. If you sprayed with a pesticide before you realized you were pregnant, don't worry about it; there is no increased incidence of miscarriage, birth defects, or childhood cancers. If your home requires repeated spraying, just be sure that the area is well ventilated after the spraying and leave your place for 8 to 12 hours afterward. The vapors and smell will have settled by then. DEET is the active ingredient in many types of creams, lotions, and sprays used as a mosquito and tick repellent. DEET is safe to use during pregnancy.

Q. *My child's school just reported an outbreak*
   of head lice. I checked her head—and mine—
   and we both have them. What can I do?

A. Don't just scratch your head. Lotions and shampoos that contain pyrethrins are safe to use during pregnancy. Pyrethrins are also used to treat scabies.

Q. *Do house pets pose a threat if
I have allergies to them?*

A. If you had an allergy to a dog or a cat before you were pregnant,
you will continue to have an allergy to these pets when you are pregnant. The same precautions should be followed—avoid contact. You
will experience the same symptoms—stuffed nose and teary eyes, for
example—but there will be no adverse effects to your fetus if this is
the extent of your symptoms. If these symptoms annoy you, you
may want to take an allergy medicine. As with all medications, they
should be avoided if possible during pregnancy, since they all have
potentially adverse effects on your developing fetus.

TRAVEL

Q. *Can I travel on a commercial
airplane during my pregnancy?*

A. Yes, airplane travel is safe for you and your fetus. If you suffer from motion sickness, there are medications you can take that
are safe to use during pregnancy. However, try to delay your trip
until the second trimester so you can avoid the use of medications,
the chance of vomiting, and the nausea that often occurs during
the first trimester.

Q. *Can I travel in a small private
plane during pregnancy?*

A. Yes. Small planes usually do not have pressurized cabins, so the
plane's altitude will be less than 7,000 feet.

Q. *Are there any special instructions for*
   me if I am planning a long trip?

A. Before you go on your trip, locate the nearest hospital where
you'll be staying and ask your doctor to recommend an obstetrician in that area should an emergency arise. If you will be gone for
several weeks, take a copy of your prenatal records with you.

   If you are embarking on a long drive or plane ride, get up and
move around every couple of hours to avoid swelling in your legs
and feet. Wear loose, comfortable clothes and dress in layers in case
you get hot and cold. Wear sandals to accommodate any swelling
that might occur in your feet during your trip, and bring heavy
socks in case your feet get cold.

Q. *Should I plan a trip near the end*
   of my pregnancy?

A. Your baby does not know your due date. He or she may come
at any time. You should not plan a trip after 34 weeks if you want
to deliver at the hospital of your choice and with the doctor of your
choice. If your trip requires travel by air, you may travel up to 36
weeks without a physician's note. If the trip is of an emergency nature, the airlines will permit travel with a medical release.

Q. *Will the airport metal detectors*
   affect my baby?

A. No. The airport metal detector you walk through will not emit
any form of harmful radiation to you or your fetus.

Q. *Should I wear seat belts when I am pregnant?*

A. Yes. Besides being effective in preventing injury to yourself and your fetus, it is also the law in many states. You should wear both the lap belt and shoulder harness. The lap belt should be worn across the thighs, under the fetus, and against your hip bones. The shoulder harness should be worn above your uterus. You may also want to place a small pillow on your lap between your uterus and the steering wheel.

Q. *Can I go on a roller coaster during my pregnancy?*

A. No. There is a theoretical concern that the g forces, quick starts and stops, and rigorous bouncing can cause a shearing force between the uterus and placenta, causing a separation called *abruptio placentae* or placental abruption. This is a disastrous event that can cause sudden bleeding and death to you and your baby. This would occur during your late second or third trimester. I am not aware of any studies linking spontaneous miscarriages to riding a roller coaster during the first trimester, but avoid them anyway; you can go on them with your child in a few years.

WORK

Q. *I have to stand during my 8-hour shift. Should I continue to work?*

A. Standing at work does not cause any pregnancy complications. Keep working.

Q. *I have a strenuous job. Should I keep working?*

A. Women who have physically strenuous jobs may continue their employment without difficulty. There is no increase in small babies or preterm labor.

Q. *I work a night shift. Should I continue working?*

A. You may want to go on days. A recent study linked pregnant night shift workers and an increased incidence of preterm labor. The risk began in the first trimester and continued throughout all trimesters.

Q. *When should I stop working?*

A. In general, you should stop working when you feel too tired to continue your usual work routine. Some women drive a long distance to and from work and may find commuting too tiring. Sometimes, especially during the last 4 weeks of your pregnancy, you may find yourself falling asleep at the wheel. In this case, either carpool or stop working. Many women can and do work up until the day they go into labor. Of course, if you have a special medical or obstetrical problem, you may be advised to stop working at any time during your pregnancy.

Q. *What is the Health Insurance Portability and Accountability Act (HIPPA)?*

A. This law protects you from losing your maternity insurance coverage if you change employment during your pregnancy. Your new job's health insurance plan must include maternity benefits.

The new plan must also cover your newborn as long as the baby is registered with the insurance company within 30 days of birth.

Q. *What is the Family Medical Leave Act (FMLA)?*

A. The FMLA is a federal law that requires all employers with fifty or more employees to permit their employees to have up to 12 weeks of unpaid leave per twelve-month period for:

- Birth of a child or adoption/foster care of a child
- Care of a spouse, child, or parent with serious health issues
- Work disability during pregnancy or postpartum

To take family leave, you must work for an employer with fifty or more employees. You must be employed at the company for at least one year and have worked at least 1,250 hours during the past twelve months.

Q. *What is the Pregnancy Discrimination Act (PDA)?*

A. The PDA is a federal law that requires employers with fifteen or more employees to treat a pregnancy-disabled employee like any other disabled employee who may temporarily need to have a lighter workload or take a leave. In addition, the PDA states that an employer cannot fire, refuse to hire, or refuse to promote a woman because she is pregnant.

SEX

Q. *Can I have sexual intercourse*
during my pregnancy?

A. Pregnancy does not mean sexual abstinence. Sexual activity will not harm the pregnancy or developing fetus in a low-risk pregnancy.

Q. *Is it safe to have sex during*
my first trimester?

A. Yes. Sexual intercourse will not cause a miscarriage. If it did, those 50 percent of you who did not plan your pregnancy and had sex would never know that you were pregnant. If sex caused miscarriages, there would be both fewer abortion clinics and fewer children in the world.

Q. *When should I avoid sex during my pregnancy?*

A. Avoid having sex during pregnancy if you have any of the following problems or conditions:

- Incompetent cervix
- Unexplained pain
- Unexplained bleeding or discharge
- Cramping
- Active genital herpes lesion in either partner
- Ruptured membranes
- Threatened abortion (pregnancy complicated by vaginal bleeding and/or cramping, causing a higher risk of spontaneous abortion) in the first trimester

- History of preterm labor (avoid sex in the latter second trimester and third trimester)
- Uncomfortable sex
- Placenta previa in the late second trimester and third trimester

Q. *Is it safe to have an orgasm during pregnancy?*

A. Yes. Orgasms will not cause miscarriages or harmful decreased blood flow to your developing fetus. However, if you have a history of preterm labor, you may want to discontinue sex and avoid orgasm at 28 to 30 weeks gestation. Orgasm may cause mild uterine contractions.

Q. *I have had two miscarriages already. Is it still safe to have sex in the first trimester?*

A. Yes. Most miscarriages (70 to 80 percent) are caused by a genetically abnormal fetus, progesterone deficiency, or immunological problems. A miscarriage that occurs after sexual activity would have occurred anyway. If you have been used to having sex on a nightly basis, this can continue without any harm to the pregnancy.

Q. *Can spotting of blood occur after having sex?*

A. This is a common occurrence. The cervix becomes very vascular, with the formation of new blood vessels on the surface, and these small blood vessels may be broken and bleed temporarily during and after sexual intercourse. There is no risk that this bleeding will cause a miscarriage.

Q. *Will my sex drive change during pregnancy?*

A. Some women feel more amorous, others less, and some women have the same desires as before they were pregnant. All of these behaviors are normal. Usually there is a decrease in sexual desire in the first trimester if you are experiencing nausea, fatigue, headaches, or breast tenderness. There also may be a decrease in sexual desire in the third trimester because of fatigue and your normal increased weight gain. Some women may have orgasms or multiple orgasms for the first time during their pregnancy owing to the higher hormone levels and increased blood flow to the pelvis.

Q. *Will my partner's sex drive change?*

A. Your partner's sexual desire may be altered by many feelings during your pregnancy: anxiety over sex harming the pregnancy or fetus, your health, and apprehension about becoming a parent and lifestyle changes. Many men are very attracted to the changing shape of their partner's body during pregnancy.

Q. *Could having sex feel uncomfortable?*

A. As your pregnancy progresses, the missionary position (man on top) may feel uncomfortable. Discuss and try different positions with your mate. Some women have a tendency for persistentent or recurrent yeast infections during pregnancy, which may cause pain during sexual intercourse.

There is an increase in blood flow to your uterus and pelvis, which can cause swelling of your vulva and vagina. Sometimes this swelling causes your vulva to enlarge and look abnormal. The swelling may also cause discomfort during sex.

Your breasts may continue to grow throughout pregnancy, and you may have to enact the "look but don't touch" rule.

Nipple stimulation during the last trimester may cause uterine contractions resulting from the release of oxytocin. This should be avoided, especially if there is a history or high risk of preterm labor or if your fetus is growth restricted.

Q. *Can sex cause preterm labor?*

A. Aside from the possible causes of preterm labor already given, there is a substance in semen called prostaglandin that may also stimulate contractions. The possibility that your partner's semen will trigger preterm labor is extremely rare. Nonetheless, it may not be advisable to have your partner ejaculate inside you if you have a risk of preterm labor.

Q. *Can my partner and I engage in oral sex when I am pregnant?*

A. Yes. This, too, is fine.

EXERCISE

Q. *Are there benefits for exercising during pregnancy?*

A. Medical research has recently pointed out that if you are physically fit before your pregnancy, you may continue to exercise during your pregnancy as long as you have no medical or obstetrical complications. Your main concern is that your fetus gets an adequate supply of oxygen. Mild aerobic activities, such as walking, jogging, swimming, cycling, yoga, and aerobics classes, are all good choices. Exercise has several health benefits:

- It improves your mood.
- It increases your energy level.
- It tones your body and increases your strength.
- It increases your endurance.
- It improves your posture.
- It improves your bowel function.
- It reduces the chance of backaches.
- It helps control how much weight you gain.
- It makes you sleep better.

In addition, if you are in good shape and perform endurance exercises, your labor may be shorter and even more tolerable. Being in good shape will provide you with stamina and endurance, which is a plus when it comes to the strenuous task of delivering a baby.

Q. *Are there exercise guidelines during pregnancy?*

A. Let your body dictate your level of exercise, and don't overdo it. If you are performing an aerobic exercise, continue as long as you can talk without feeling breathless. Avoid floor exercises on your back after 20 weeks, and use a pillow to wedge yourself to the side. Stop exercising if you experience any of the following:

- Vaginal bleeding
- Dizziness

- Chest pain
- Headache
- Preterm labor
- Decreased fetal movement
- Leakage of amniotic fluid

Q. *Who shouldn't exercise when pregnant?*

A. Avoid exercising if:

- You have serious heart disease or lung disease
- You have severe anemia
- You are seriously underweight or overweight
- You have poorly controlled diabetes, hypertension, seizure disorder, or thyroid disorder
- You have a history of incompetent cervix
- You are having multiple births and are in the second trimester
- You have placenta previa and are in the third trimester
- You are experiencing preterm labor during your current pregnancy
- You have a low-birth-weight pregnancy

Q. *I'm in great shape. Can I continue to exercise at my present level?*

A. Nature has its ways of curtailing your activities! For instance, during the first 13 weeks of pregnancy, at least 50 percent of women experience nausea and vomiting. During the next 27 weeks, hormonal changes may cause fatigue and lack of motivation. Even if you don't suffer these changes, you should decrease your level of training to adapt to your weight gain, particularly from the fifth month on. The extra weight alone will make your normal workout more difficult.

Q. *I was a runner before pregnancy.*
Can I still run during pregnancy?

A. You can continue to run during pregnancy. Remember to keep well hydrated, and buy new running shoes as your feet expand during pregnancy.

Q. *Is it safe to begin an exercise program*
once I become pregnant if I've
been sedentary up to this point?

A. Yes, you can begin an exercise program, but with some limitations. For instance, now is not the time to strive to get into "world-class" shape. Start your exercise routine slowly. Begin by exercising 5 minutes the first day, and add 5 minutes every day if you can until you are exercising 30 to 60 minutes a day.

Q. *Can I cycle during my pregnancy?*

A. Cycling is another good aerobic form of exercise to continue or start during pregnancy. Your body weight and joints are supported. In the latter part of your pregnancy, if your center of balance has shifted and you feel uneasy about riding, cycle on a stationary bike. If your big belly starts to get in the way of pedaling or if your back can't tolerate cycling in the upright position, use a recumbent bike.

Q. *Can I use an elliptical machine when I am pregnant?*

A. These machines offer a great low-impact form of aerobic exercise. You can use this machine throughout pregnancy.

Q. *Can I do yoga during pregnancy?*

A. You may continue your yoga classes or start a pregnancy yoga class. Yoga is supposed to be relaxing and relieve your stress. Avoid lying flat on your back during your third trimester if this makes you dizzy. Do not take Bikram-style "hot yoga" classes; you don't want to get overheated.

Q. *Can I take an aerobics class during pregnancy?*

A. You can continue to take your aerobics classes during pregnancy. I would alter the routine if it is a high-impact class; your joints will thank you. If you are a beginner to aerobics, take a pregnancy class.

Q. *Can I weight train during pregnancy?*

A. Yes. The goal of weight training during pregnancy is to improve your muscle tone. The exercises should be done with low weights and high repetitions. This will avoid undue strain and pressure on your joints. Avoid bench work. Work on your core.

Q. *Must I stop exercising during my last month of pregnancy?*

A. Not unless your doctor suggests you do so because of obstetrical complications. However, it would be advisable to cut back if you experience back problems, swelling of your extremities, lack of balance, or extreme fatigue or discomfort because of weight gain. If you experience none of these problems, then mild exercise is perfectly all right until you go into labor.

Q. *How will I know if I am exercising too much?*

A. If you are exercising and eating a balanced diet but do not gain the prescribed 20 to 30 pounds, you may be exercising too much and too hard. I recommend that you consult your doctor to discuss modifying your exercise program and caloric intake. Physically fit women will lose their weight gain within the first three months after giving birth.

Q. *What activities should I avoid when I'm pregnant?*

A. Avoid sports such as snow skiing and waterskiing, rollerblading, mountain climbing, downhill mountain biking, and horseback riding. Also avoid sports in which you are intensely competitive and which may cause injury to you or your fetus, such as tennis, softball, or soccer, especially in your second and third trimesters. Your joints and ligaments become particularly lax during pregnancy as a result of hormonal changes, and they don't give you the support and stability necessary to safely perform some activities.

Q. *Can I go scuba diving during my pregnancy?*

A. Pregnant women should not scuba dive. The fetus cannot tolerate the decompression that occurs when a scuba diver surfaces.

There is an increased risk of miscarriages, birth defects, preterm delivery, low-birth-weight babies, and stillbirths.

Q. *Is swimming a good exercise during pregnancy?*

A. Swimming is one of the best exercises for pregnant women. You are not exerting any pressure on your joints, and you don't have to worry about your balance. You will enjoy a great cardiovascular workout without overheating.

Q. *Can I swim in a lake or river during my pregnancy?*

A. Swimming in natural waters such as lakes, rivers, or streams may expose you and your fetus to potential risk. Leptospirosis, a bacterial disease, has become endemic in many areas of the United States. Infection follows contact through broken skin, such as cracks in the skin between toes, while swimming in a stream contaminated by infected rodent or dog urine. The resulting illness may cause miscarriage or preterm labor. Giardiasis and amebiasis are two parasitic infections that may be contracted by swimming in or drinking from contaminated water from streams or ponds. Giardiasis causes mild to severe painful diarrhea but no untoward effects to the pregnancy or fetus. Amebiasis may cause a miscarriage or maternal death.

Q. *Is it safe to swim in a pool during my pregnancy?*

A. As long as the water has been adequately chlorinated and the pH has been properly maintained, swimming in a public pool is considered safe during pregnancy, although swimmers must comply with proper hygienic conduct. There are some viral infections that may be transmitted from swimming in contaminated pool water. There is usually a rise in enterovirus infections during the summertime, and women in their third trimester should avoid swimming if an epidemic is in the area. Infection with these viruses could cause a life-threatening infection in the fetus. Hepatitis A may be transmitted by contact with a contaminated pool. Most cases of infection during pregnancy are asymptomatic.

There is no risk of contracting a sexually transmitted disease from pool water, although herpes simplex and human papillomavirus may be contracted from surfaces around the pool. HIV is not spread in public swimming pool water.

CHAPTER 6

Drugs and Medications

ALCOHOL

Q. *Can I drink alcohol when
I am pregnant?*

A. The Surgeon General advises all pregnant women not to drink alcohol. This admonition is also found in the Bible: "Behold, thou shalt conceive, and bear a son, and now drink no wine or strong drink. . . ." (Judges 13:7).

The placenta does not act as a barrier for alcohol. Any alcohol you drink will get into your developing baby's bloodstream within minutes of drinking and will be in the same concentration as in your own. Before you have a drink just think whether you would put even a little beer or wine into your baby's bottle.

Q. *What are the effects to
my pregnancy if I drink?*

A. The risk of miscarriage is twice as high if you drink only one ounce of absolute alcohol (AA) as rarely as twice a week. That is four glasses of wine per week. Women who drink more that 1½ ounces of absolute alcohol a day will have an increased risk of premature labor or postterm pregnancy (lasting more than 42 weeks).

Q. *What are the effects of
alcohol on my baby?*

A. The effects on your baby have been collectively termed fetal alcohol spectrum disorders (FASD). These disorders can be manifested as birth defects, neurological problems, and mental disabilities. The severity of the disorders is based on the amount of alcohol you drink each day, constant binge drinking, and your genetic composition. These disorders and the effects of alcohol on your fetus are irreversible. About 40,000 babies a year are born with FASD. That is about 1 percent of babies born every year.

Q. *What is fetal alcohol syndrome?*

A. Fetal alcohol syndrome (FAS) usually occurs in babies whose mothers drank heavily throughout the pregnancy. Binge drinking (more that five drinks at a time consistently or more than seven alcoholic beverages a week) will put your baby at greatest risk for FAS. The sad part is that these babies look so cute. They have small heads, eyes, and an upturned nose. The babies have thin lips without a philtrum (the shallow groove running down from the center of the upper lip to the nose) and flat cheeks. Sadly, these appealing features fade as the baby matures. The most unfortunate alcohol-related effects include:

Poor sucking/nursing
Poor sleep patterns
Hyperactive behavior
Poor coordination
Developmental delays in speech and learning
Low IQ

Poor memory
Poor reasoning skills
Low attention span
Impaired judgment
Poor impulse control
Vision and hearing problems
Poor communication skills
Problems getting along with others

The birth defects can include heart, eye, ear, kidney, and bone abnormalities. These defects are actually abnormal growth patterns caused by the alcohol destroying cells in the developing organs. If your drinking average is one alcoholic beverage per day, your child will develop FAS. Alcohol is the most common known cause of mental retardation that is 100 percent preventable by not consuming alcohol during pregnancy.

Q. *What is partial fetal alcohol syndrome?*

A. The syndrome results in the baby having the characteristic face of FAS babies and either growth or learning and behavioral problems.

Q. *What is alcohol-related neurodevelopmental disorder?*

A. The babies have learning and/or behavioral disorders, but do not have the typical facial features or growth delays.

Q. *What are alcohol-related birth defects?*

A. These babies have only the birth defects listing previously, without the typical face or learning problems.

Q. *Before I knew I was pregnant, I would*
drink a glass of wine with dinner.
How will this affect my baby?

A. There is no safe amount of alcohol consumption during pregnancy. The effects of drinking alcohol during early pregnancy are unknown. If you were not consistently binge drinking or drinking heavily (more than seven drinks a week), the risks to your baby will be minimal to none. The most important step for you to take is to stop drinking now. The effects of alcohol on the fetus are variable. Some women may drink fairly heavily and their babies do not seem to be affected, while other babies may be affected with less alcohol abuse.

Q. *How common is drinking alcohol*
in the beginning of pregnancy?

A. Fairly common. Consider this: About 50 percent of women up to age 30 drink regularly, and 50 percent of pregnancies are unintended. Therefore, at least 25 percent of women are unknowingly drinking alcohol at the beginning of their pregnancies.

CIGARETTES AND ILLICIT DRUGS

Q. *What are the possible complications*
of smoking on my pregnancy?

A. Possible complications include the following:

- Abruptio placentae (premature separation of the placenta) is 1½ times more common in smokers because of necrotic areas in the placenta.

- Placenta previa (implantation of the placenta low in the uterus, covering or partially covering the opening of the cervix) is twice as common in smokers as in nonsmokers.
- Preterm premature rupture of the membranes and term premature rupture of the membranes are both twice as common in smokers.
- Preterm births are 20 percent more common in smokers.
- The perinatal death rate in babaies born to smokers is increased by 150 percent.

Women who smoke have babies that smoke. This causes the babies to receive less oxygen and food, so these babies are starved and are smaller babies. This is dose dependent. The more you smoke, the smaller your baby. The greatest decrease in weight is about 7 ounces. These children may also lag behind in learning ability by almost six months. There is also a much higher incidence of SIDS (sudden infant death syndrome). Moreover, these children grow up with an increased incidence of asthma, colic, respiratory illnesses, middle ear infections, impaired lung function, and childhood obesity.

Q. *Will secondhand smoke affect my pregnancy?*

A. Yes. If you are in an environment where you are constantly exposed to secondhand smoke, your baby can have low birth weight and lung disorders.

Q. *How can I stop smoking?*

A. Asking this question is a fine beginning. Ask for help from your OB, family doctor, family members, and partner. If your partner also smokes, ask him to also be your "quitting buddy."

Great Start is a national pregnancy-specific hotline. The phone number is 1-866-66-START.

You can also try behavioral therapy, hypnosis, acupuncture, or medical therapy. Online resources include: helppregnantsmokersquit.org/quit/toll_free.asp and smokefreefamilies.org.

Q. *Can I use a nicotine substitute to help me stop smoking during my pregnancy?*

A. If you have not been successful using the above support systems, you can use nicotine replacement therapy. Intermittent therapy should be used. Try nicotine gum or inhalers first. You can use the nicotine patch during the day, removing it at bedtime. Nicotine replacement therapy can also be used during lactation. The package inserts on these patches suggest that pregnant women not use these devices unless advised to do so by their physicians because of the danger that nicotine poses to the developing fetus. However, nicotine is not the only toxin in cigarette smoke, and substitution of the patch will certainly decrease fetal exposure to carbon monoxide and other toxins. If you would like to stop smoking during your pregnancy and have failed on your own, the use of a nicotine patch is a reasonable option you should ask your doctor about.

Q. *What are the effects of marijuana smoking during pregnancy?*

A. The same effects as for cigarette smoking have been demonstrated for marijuana smoking during pregnancy. In addition, there seems to be an increased risk of prematurity, precipitous (fast) labor, and meconium passage (a sign of fetal distress). No increased incidence of malformations in the fetus due to marijuana has been shown. However, babies born to women who are marijuana smokers have problems responding to environmental stimuli and may have tremors. These changes seem to resolve by the end of the first month of life.

Q. *I smoked marijuana before I knew*
I was pregnant. Is my baby okay?

A. There seem to be no effects on your baby if you smoked a few times in the first trimester.

CAFFEINE

Q. *Will drinking products containing*
caffeine cause a miscarriage?

A. Caffeine crosses the placenta and may stimulate your baby. In one study in which women drank up to 3 cups of coffee a day, there was no increased incidence of miscarriage. This was equal to 300 milligrams of caffeine per day. This was the study that the FDA utilized to formulate their recommendations on caffeine usage during pregnancy: moderate use of caffeine (300 milligrams a day) is safe throughout pregnancy.

Q. *How does caffeine affect my pregnancy?*

A. Caffeine is not an agent that causes birth defects in humans. Caffeine consumption alone did not cause a decrease in birth weight or the development of fetal growth restriction (FGR) in several studies. However, the heaviest caffeine users in these studies (more than 300 milligrams a day) also were more likely to smoke and/or drink alcohol. These pregnancies were complicated by an increased risk of miscarriage and low-birth-weight babies.

Q. *How much caffeine can*
I safely consume each day?

A. A moderate amount of caffeine consumption would be up to 300 milligrams a day.

MEDICATIONS

Q. *Before I knew that I was pregnant, I took a*
particular medication. What will this do to my baby?

A. Exposure to certain medicines or drugs probably accounts for 2 to 3 percent of all birth defects. The fetus is most sensitive to a drug's effects during the period when its organs are developing. This takes place from the 31st to the 71st day after your last menstrual period. Any medicine or drug ingested before this time has an all-or-none effect: either the fetus survives without birth defects or it does not survive at all. At least 50 percent of pregnant moms know that they are pregnant before day 31.

Q. *I took my birth control pills for*
some time before I realized I was pregnant.
Will my baby have a birth defect?

A. No. A woman who has taken oral contraceptives during her pregnancy will not increase her risk of major congenital malformations over the normal baseline rate of 2 to 3 percent. Of course, if you find out you are pregnant while taking the pill, there is no reason to continue taking it.

Q. *I became pregnant while using an intrauterine device (IUD). What effect will this have on my pregnancy?*

A. There is no evidence that a pregnancy with an IUD in place will cause a congenital anomaly. Pregnancies with an IUD are associated with an increased frequency of spontaneous miscarriages. If the IUD can be removed easily, this should be done. There is also an increased frequency of tubal (ectopic) pregnancies when pregnancies occur during IUD use, so an early ultrasound should be performed to confirm the location of your pregnancy.

Q. *I became pregnant while using a vaginal spermicide. Will my baby have an increased incidence of birth defects?*

A. There is no increase in the risk of congenital malformations in babies born to women who became pregnant while using vaginal spermicides or who use vaginal spermicides during the course of their pregnancy.

Q. *I took Provera to bring on my period, but I was pregnant. What are the effects on my baby?*

A. Provera is a synthetic form of progesterone and was at one time thought to cause developmental malformations. This has since been found to be untrue. The inadvertent use of Provera will not cause a birth defect.

Q. *Is it safe to take over-the-counter*
  medicines when I am pregnant?

A. A general rule is: do not take any medicine, prescription or nonprescription, without the consent of your doctor. Another general rule is: assume that all medicines are potentially harmful to your developing fetus. A third general rule is: only take a medicine whose benefit will far outweigh its potential risk to mother and fetus. Only your doctor can make that decision.

Despite the cautions to avoid drugs and the indiscriminate ingestion of medicine, recent surveys have found the average pregnant woman takes up to five drugs or medicines during her pregnancy that contain nine different pharmacological agents. The most common are prenatal vitamins, iron supplements, antacids, antiemetics (antinausea medicines), analgesics, and antihistamines.

Q. *What can I use for the treatment of*
  diarrhea during pregnancy?

A. Kaopectate should be tried first. Kaopectate does not get absorbed by your intestines and therefore does not get into your bloodstream. Immodium can safely be used after your 10th week. Pepto-Bismol does not cause birth defects but releases a compound that could, on rare occasions, cause bleeding problems.

Q. *I used aspirin in my first trimester*
  before I realized I was pregnant.
  Did I harm my baby?

A. The use of aspirin at the beginning of pregnancy is fairly common. The aspirin is usually taken alone or in combination with cold, flu, or headache preparations. Numerous studies have been conducted, and the combined reports link aspirin use with a birth defect called *gastroschisis*. The risk is 1 in 15,000. If you are worried, a second-trimester ultrasound can detect if the intestines are floating free in the amniotic cavity as a result of a hole in the baby's abdomen.

Q. *Can I use adult aspirin in the second and third trimesters?*

A. The use of regular-dose (325-milligram) aspirin may cause bleeding in you and your newborn if taken within a week of delivery. Aspirin may also cause premature closure of blood vessels around the heart, causing problems with your baby's circulation at birth. If you want to take an aspirin for a headache, try lying down and relaxing first. Remember, too, that aspirin is found in many over-the-counter cold and allergy medicines.

Q. *Can I use products containing ibuprofen during pregnancy?*

A. Ibuprofen may also be weakly linked to gastroschisis if taken in the first trimester. Like aspirin, ibuprofen may cause excessive bleeding in you, causing postpartum hemorrhage or bleeding problems with your baby at the time of delivery if used at term. Theoretically, ibuprofen may prolong your pregnancy if used at term; medications similar to ibuprofen are now being used to stop preterm labor. Ibuprofen can also decrease your baby's kidney function and cause *oligohydramnios*, a decreased amount of amniotic fluid. Ibuprofen is even more potent than aspirin in constricting the blood vessels around the heart, causing circulatory difficulties at birth. For these reasons, ibuprofen should not be used near the time of delivery.

Q. *Can I take acetaminophen (Tylenol, Datril, Panadol) during pregnancy?*

A. There is no evidence that acetaminophen causes birth defects, and it's not toxic to the newborn. Acetaminophen is the preferred medication to take during pregnancy for headaches, fever, or body or muscle aches. The maximum amount of acetaminophen used per day should not exceed 4,000 milligrams.

Q. *Can I use pseudoephedrine during my pregnancy?*

A. Pseudoephedrine is a decongestant that may provide symptomatic relief of rhinitis (runny nose) and sinusitis. According to some large studies, there is probably no increased incidence of birth defects from the use of decongestants during pregnancy, but try to limit their use to the second or third trimester. Try using a hot or cold humidifier and a saline nasal spray to help clear secretions, and drink plenty of fluids.

Q. *Can I use antihistamines during pregnancy?*

A. Antihistamines are used to relieve rhinitis, watery eyes, and itching. Once again, large studies have not shown increased incidence of birth defects from the use of antihistamines during pregnancy. If you can, use chlorpheniramine or tripelennamine during the first trimester. You may use cetirizine or loratadine in the second and third trimesters.

Q. *Can I use a cough suppressant
during pregnancy?*

A. Yes. Dextromethorphan, the most commonly used nonprescription cough medicine, has been shown safe to use throughout pregnancy.

Q. *Can I use an expectorant
during pregnancy?*

A. Expectorants relieve dry coughs by loosening up the thick secretions so that they may be removed naturally by coughing. Guaifenesin is the most frequently used expectorant found in cold preparations and may be used throughout pregnancy without an increase in congenital malformations.

Q. *Can I use an acne preparation
containing benzoyl peroxide?*

A. Yes. Benzoyl peroxide is a bactericidal agent that will act on the bacteria (*Propione bacterium*) that causes acne. Only minute amounts of this medication are absorbed through the skin and are then excreted by your kidneys.

Q. *Which medicines are known
to have effects on the fetus?*

A. Here is a list of medicines and their effects on the fetus:

- Accutane—birth defects
- Alcohol—birth defects

- Coumadin—birth defects
- DES—birth defects
- Dilantin—birth defects
- Methotrexate—birth defects
- Methyl mercury—nerve damage, FGR (fetal growth restriction)
- Sulfa at term—jaundice
- Testosterone—masculinization
- Tetracycline—discoloration of teeth, decreased bone growth
- Thalidomide—birth defects
- Tobacco—prematurity, IUGR (intrauterine growth retardation), birth defects
- Vaccinations (some)—birth defects
- Vitamins (some, in excess)—birth defects

SELECTIVE SERATONIN REUPTAKE INHIBITORS (SSRI)

Q. *I am on an SSRI and I am planning to get pregnant in the near future. What should I do?*

A. Go to the physician who placed you on the SSRI for a consult. Consult with your psychologist as well if you have one. Studies have shown that if you have mild depression, treatment with either an SSRI or psychotherapy is equally effective. Therefore, if you think that you may have mild depression and you are on an SSRI, seek out a psychotherapist and wean yourself off the SSRI. If you have moderate depression, stay on your SSRI.

Q. *I am taking an SSRI and just found out that I am pregnant. What should I do?*

A. Most large studies have shown that it is safe to take SSRIs throughout pregnancy. One recent study showed a slight increase in birth defects with Paxil. Never abruptly discontinue your SSRI. This can cause a sudden worsening in your emotional state.

Q. *Which SSRIs are safe to take during pregnancy?*

A. Celexa, Lexapro, Prozac, and Zoloft are all considered safe.

X-RAYS AND MRI

Q. *I had some X-rays performed before I realized that I was pregnant. What will happen to my baby?*

A. The risk to the fetus of any birth defect is extremely low. Some studies have reported an increased likelihood of childhood leukemia in the offspring of women exposed to X-rays during pregnancy. This risk increases the number of leukemia cases from 2 per 6,000 to 3 per 6,000, a very small increase compared with the risk of childhood leukemia to a newborn whose sibling has childhood leukemia (1 per 720). The risk of birth defects to the fetus increases after a radiation exposure of from 5 to 10 rads (radiation absorbed doses). Most X-ray studies will not expose the fetus to this degree of risk and if ordered by your doctor are necessary for your health and usually on an emergency basis. Of course, X-rays that can be avoided until after pregnancy should be delayed.

Q. *How much radiation from X-rays is dangerous to my baby?*

A. Generally, radiation exposure from a single diagnostic procedure does not result in any harmful effects. Exposure to the fetus of 5 rads or less is safe and has not been observed to cause birth defects, miscarriages, or growth restriction (low birth weight).

Q. *I had a CT scan of my pelvis/abdomen or spine. Did I get too much radiation?*

A. No. Your baby was exposed to only 3.5 rads.

Q. *I had a barium enema before I knew I was pregnant. How much radiation did I receive?*

A. About 2 to 4 rads, depending on the number of X-rays taken.

Q. *I had a hysterosalpingogram and I was pregnant. Did I cause a miscarriage?*

A. No, this procedure will not cause you to miscarry, and the fetus only received 50 millirads.

Q. *I am pregnant. I felt a lump in my breast and need a mammogram. How much radiation exposure will my baby get?*

A. Your fetus will get only 7 to 20 millirads.

Q. *I need a special nuclear scan to determine if I have a pulmonary embolus (blood clot in the lung). Is this safe to do?*

A. Yes. The fetal exposure is only 50 millirads.

Q. *I had an MRI before I knew I was pregnant. Will this affect my fetus?*

A. No. Magnetic resonance imaging does not use ionizing radiation, but instead uses a magnetic field. There is no indication that an MRI study will pose harm to your fetus.

Q. *What are the possible complications of using herbal medicines during pregnancy?*

A. Herbal medicines are natural medicines or drugs in their most basic form. The active ingredients in these herbs possess the same chemicals found in many prescription medicines. These herbs can therefore have the same ability to treat certain disorders and the same ability to cause side effects. Possible complications include:

- Miscarriage
- Birth defects
- Kidney and liver damage
- Bleeding problems
- Preterm labor
- Hyperstimulation of the uterus, causing dangerous hypoxia (low oxygen) in your baby
- Lead poisoning in your baby
- Mercury poisoning in your baby

Q. *Can I drink herbal tea during my pregnancy?*

A. The FDA would rather you not drink most herbal teas during pregnancy and while breast-feeding. Red raspberry leaf tea, called the "pregnancy" tea, has been used to treat morning sickness, prevent miscarriages, induce labor, shorten labor, and relieve the pain of labor. This tea has not proved to be effective in doing any of these things, but it does contain vitamins and iron and does not appear to have any side effects to mom or baby. It is unknown, however, whether or not it can cause birth defects.

CHAPTER 7

Special Tests

Q. *What is the extended AFP test or AFP quad test?*

A. The alpha-fetoprotein (AFP) quadruple blood test measures four markers in your blood that increase the ability to detect a Down syndrome pregnancy, neural tube defects (NTDs), Smith-Lemli-Opitz syndrome, trisomy 18, and an increased risk of certain pregnancy complications, such as preterm labor, low-birth-weight babies, and stillborns. This blood test is a screening test for these abnormalities and not a diagnostic test. The results of the test will indicate whether you will be at greater risk of having a baby with a birth defect or a pregnancy complication.

Q. *When do I take the AFP quad test?*

A. The test is performed between the 15th and 20th week of your pregnancy. The best time to take the test is during your 16th to 17th week.

Q. *What is the meaning of a positive low AFP quad screen?*

A. Remember that this test is a screening test and not a diagnostic test. Therefore, most positive results are false positives. The most likely explanation for a positive result is a normal variation in blood levels. It is also possible that your pregnancy is further along or not as far along as you thought, or you may have a twin or multiple pregnancy. It may also mean that your risk for having a pregnancy complication or a baby with a birth defect is higher. Listen to your doctor's full explanation of the results. Many women start crying as soon as they hear that the test result is positive; they think the worst—that their baby has a birth defect or that their pregnancy will end in disaster. This is rarely the case. Your doctor will explain that your risk of having a baby with Down syndrome, for example, is greater than 1 in190, which is the cutoff for your test. For example, my son's result came back as 1 in 67, which meant that his risk of being born with Down syndrome was 1.5 percent and 66 out of 67 babies born with this risk would not have Down syndrome (he did not).

Q. *If the AFP is high; does that mean*
that my baby has a neural tube defect?

A. No. The incidence of neural tube defects is 1 or 2 per 1,000 pregnancies. This test will be positive in 5 out of 100 pregnancies. Therefore, if you have a positive test result, you will have to undergo additional tests. It is possible that you are further along in your pregnancy or that you are carrying twins. This test will detect all cases of anencephaly and approximately 80 percent of spina bifida cases.

Q. *What will be the next step if
I have a positive test result?*

A. The first step should be an ultrasound exam to confirm your
pregnancy dates. If the dating is incorrect, this information will be
given to the laboratory, and your results will be recalculated. If the
results now come back in the normal range, there is nothing more
to do. If your gestational dates are correct, your doctor will discuss
the other prenatal tests that may be performed. You may have genetic counseling, an ultrasound performed by a perinatologist, and
an amniocentesis if you so desire.

Q. *Do I have to take the AFP quad screen test?*

A. No. This is a voluntary blood test. The extended AFP or quad
test is a state-run test. The cost of the test in California is $105. If
you have maternity coverage with your health insurance plan, the
cost will be covered less your deductible or co-pay. The cost of any
and all diagnostic services—genetic counseling, ultrasound, and
amniocentesis (if performed)—at a state-approved Prenatal Diagnosis Center will be paid by the state.

Q. *Why should I take the AFP quad screen?*

A. The quad test is considered a routine procedure that is nonin-
vasive. A negative result is reassuring that your pregnancy is low risk
for certain birth defects and pregnancy complications. The test can
be used in combination with the nuchal translucency test with biochemical markers and a second-trimester ultrasound in women over
thirty-five to detect Down syndrome without invasive tests (CVS
or amniocentesis). The tests may be useful to screen for certain

anomalies if you have a family history for a birth defect. If you have a history of a previous pregnancy complication, such as preterm labor, a negative result with this test will be reassuring. If you have diabetes, you are at greater risks for complications that can be screened by this test. If you had a first-trimester viral infection or exposure to potentially harmful medicines, drugs, or high levels of radiation, the quad test can be useful to rule out possible complications.

Q. *Are any new tests available for detecting a chromosomal abnormality?*

A. Researchers are constantly working on new ways to detect chromosomal abnormalities. One promising new test is the separation of fetal cells from the maternal blood. This is being done in the first trimester, and the fetal cells may then be examined for a variety of abnormalities. Once this assay is perfected, many anomalies will be screened for by a simple blood test.

Q. *What additional tests will I take?*

A. An amniocentesis and ultrasound will be performed by a perinatologist. This test may detect a neural tube defect, kidney defects, intestinal problems, neck or spinal tumors, or a multiple pregnancy.

Q. *My AFP came back high, I had an ultrasound performed by the perinatologist, and my fetus does not have a neural tube defect. Is everything all right now?*

A. Possibly. An elevated AFP level is also associated with fetal growth restriction (FGR), stillborns, placenta accreta (abnormal adherence of the placenta to the uterus), preterm labor, labor, premature rupture of the chorioamniotic membranes, and low level of amniotic fluid (oligohydramnios) in the third trimester. Weekly nonstress tests and ultrasounds should be performed to monitor your fetus in the third trimester.

Q. *What is a neural tube defect?*

A. The neural tube is formed by the 6th week of your pregnancy. The neural tube forms from the top of your baby's head to the bottom of its spine. A neural tube defect is a birth defect in the spine or skull of your fetus resulting in either anencephaly (the top of the skull is missing, as is most of the brain) or spina bifida (part of the bones in the spine are not formed, allowing the spinal column to protrude out the back of the baby). As many as 95 percent of children born with neural tube defects are born to couples with no family history of these defects.

Q. *If my AFP quad test came back positive for a neural tube defect, what is my risk of having a baby with a neural tube defect?*

A. Only 2 percent of positive high AFP results will have a baby affected with a neural tube defect.

Q. *How common are neural tube defects?*

A. Not common at all. About 4,000 fetuses in the United States are affected each year, and about 1,300 of these fetuses either spontaneously abort or the parents choose to electively abort.

Q. *Are these problems serious?*

A. Babies born with anencephaly die within 48 hours of birth.
There are varying degrees of spina bifida, depending on the size of
the opening, where the defect is located, and if the nerves are covered with skin. Most babies born with spina bifida are paralyzed or
very weak from the waist down, cannot control their bladder or
bowels, and may eventually develop hydrocephalus (water on the
brain). Most babies have a normal IQ unless they develop hydrocephalus that goes untreated.

Q. *My ultrasound showed that I*
have a baby with spina bifida.
What are my options?

A. There are special centers throughout the United States that are
performing fetal surgery to correct spina bifida. You can contact
support groups and plan for care of a special-needs child. You may
decide not to continue your pregnancy.

Q. *How can I prevent my baby from*
having a neural tube defect?

A. Studies in the United States and other countries have shown
that the addition of low doses of supplemental folic acid may prevent many of the first-time occurrences of neural tube defects. Ac-
cordingly, the U.S. Public Health Service has recommended that all
women of childbearing age who are capable of becoming pregnant
take a vitamin supplement containing 0.4 milligram (400 micrograms) of folic acid for at least one month prior to conception and
for the first 6 weeks of the pregnancy. In addition, you should eat

a well-balanced diet with foods rich in folic acid, such as green leafy vegetables, citrus fruits, liver, and breakfast cereals fortified with folic acid. This is important because 90 percent of babies born with neural tube defects are born to couples without a family history of neural tube defects or risk factors.

Q. *What are the risk factors for having a baby with a neural tube defect?*

A. Risk factors include the following:

- Previous pregnancy with a neural tube defect (risk increases to 2 percent)
- Pregnant with poorly controlled insulin-dependent diabetes
- Use of certain antiseizure medicines during the first trimester
- Excessive obesity
- High prolonged fever or high core temperatures by recurrent hot tub or sauna use
- By race—Hispanics, whites, Afro-Americans, Asians (in descending order of risk)

Q. *What is Smith-Lemli-Opitz Syndrome?*

A. This is an autosomal recessive disorder like cystic fibrosis. The incidence is 1 in 20,000 births. If both mother and father are carriers, they will have a 25 percent chance of having an affected baby. These babies have a defect in their cholesterol metabolism that causes multiple birth defects and mental retardation.

ULTRASOUND

Q. *What is an ultrasound machine?*

A. An ultrasound machine uses high-frequency sound waves (which cannot be heard) to produce a picture of the fetus. These sound waves are produced by a transducer, a handheld instrument that is placed over your abdomen or in your vagina. The waves bounce off the organs and tissues of the fetus and placenta and are picked up by the transducer and translated into a picture by a computer onto a video screen. With the ultrasound, many malformations can be detected, but not all. The age of the fetus can be ascertained by measuring the fetal head, abdomen, and thigh bone; the position and age of the placenta can be determined; the amount of amniotic fluid can be measured; and the sex of your baby and the number of fetuses may be seen. The image of your baby may be hard for you to visualize, so ask your doctor to point out what he or she sees.

Q. *Is it necessary to perform an ultrasound during my pregnancy?*

A. Some doctors perform one or two ultrasounds routinely during a pregnancy, other doctors only for specific indications. Ask your doctor about his or her practice.

Q. *How is an ultrasound exam performed?*

A. There are two methods of performing an ultrasound exam, depending on the gestational age of your fetus. If your pregnancy is 12 weeks or less, a vaginal probe ultrasound is performed. The vaginal probe is a thin instrument that is placed in your vagina that will give your doctor a clear picture of your pregnancy, uterus, tubes, and ovaries. The probe is more comfortable than a pelvic or speculum exam. You do not need a full bladder for this procedure. An abdominal ultrasound exam is performed after 12 weeks gestation. A full bladder may be required to obtain a clear picture. A special gel will be placed on your abdomen to further enhance the quality of the ultrasound picture.

Q. *Is ultrasound harmful to my baby?*

A. Studies over the past thirty-five years have shown no ill effects, either physical or developmental, to the fetus. The doptone, the device your doctor uses to listen to the fetal heart tones, and the external fetal monitor used during labor to record the fetal heart tones also employ ultrasound waves and are also safe to use during pregnancy.

Q. *Why would I have an ultrasound in the first trimester?*

A. During the first trimester, you might have an ultrasound for any of these reasons:

- To see a heartbeat and confirm viability
- To confirm the location of the pregnancy in the uterus and not in the tube (ectopic pregnancy)
- To determine the gestational age of your baby if you are unsure of the date of your last menstrual period or if on pelvic exam your uterine size does not match your dates
- To determine if you have an ovarian cyst or uterine

fibroid, previously detected by your doctor on a
pelvic exam
- To determine if you have a multiple gestation if you had
assisted reproduction to become pregnant
- To determine if you have a multiple gestation if your
uterine size was larger than your dates would indicate
as assessed by your doctor
- To determine the risk of Down syndrome by measuring
for nuchal translucency and observe for the presence or
absence of the nasal bone
- To determine the location of the placenta and assist in
performing CVS

Q. *Why would I have an ultrasound*
during my second trimester?

A. During the second trimester, you might have an ultrasound
for any of these reasons:

- To determine congenital anomalies, such as Down syndrome
- To determine if there are structural defects, such as
anencephaly
- To determine the location of the placenta
- To determine if your dates are correct
- To determine proper fetal growth
- To determine size of uterine fibroids or ovarian cysts
- To determine the amount of amniotic fluid
- To determine the number of vessels and insertion of
the umbilical cord
- To determine the location of the placenta, fetus, and
cord when performing an amniocentesis

- To determine the cause of vaginal bleeding
- To determine the cause of pelvic pain
- To determine the length of the cervix for possible incompetent cervix
- To determine the validity of an abnormal AFP quad screen
- To determine the length of the cervix in patients at risk for preterm labor
- To determine fetal viability if the baby's heartbeat is not heard with the doptone
- To determine the gender of your baby

Q. *Why would I have an ultrasound in my third trimester?*

A. During the third trimester, you might have an ultrasound for any of these reasons:

- To determine or verify the gender of your baby
- To determine the location of the placenta if previously noted to be a placenta previa or low lying
- To determine fetal growth if the fundal height measurement was too big or too small
- To determine the quantity of amniotic fluid if the fundal height measurement was too big or too small
- To determine fetal growth
- To determine cervical length and the presence of funneling in patients at risk for preterm labor
- To determine the position of your baby for breech presentation
- To determine the cause of vaginal bleeding
- To determine the growth of babies in a multiple gestation

- To determine the well-being of your baby by performing a biophysical profile
- To determine fetal maturity by performing an amniocentesis before 37 weeks gestation
- To determine fetal size if macrosomia is suspected and a cesarean section is being contemplated for the mode of delivery

Q. *We did not see a heartbeat on my first ultrasound at 7 weeks. Should I be concerned?*

A. If you had a positive pregnancy test at least 2 weeks before the exam, fetal heart motion should be observed. If you can see a yolk sac and a fetus measuring at least 6 millimeters, a fetal heart beat should be seen.

Q. *When is the best time to confirm the age of my baby?*

A. The best time to date your pregnancy is between 9 and 12 weeks.

Q. *My doctor will only do two ultrasounds during my pregnancy. Is that normal?7*

A. Every doctor has his or her own routine for caring for a low-risk pregnancy. Some doctors will only perform two ultrasounds; others may schedule ultrasounds every two months. If you are concerned about the health of your baby or just need reassurance, ask your doctor to schedule an ultrasound for you.

Q. *Should I get a nonmedical ultrasound?*

A. Commercial, or boutique, ultrasound companies offering nonmedical ultrasounds for DVD souvenirs are not sanctioned by the FDA. In fact, using an ultrasound without a doctor's order may be unlawful.

Q. *What are choroid plexus cysts?*

A. These are cysts that may be found in the baby's brain. They are found in 1 to 3 percent of all babies during a second-trimester ultrasound. They usually disappear by 24 weeks and cause no problem. An isolated choroid plexus cyst is normal.

Q. *My second-trimester ultrasound showed that my baby has only two umbilical vessels instead of three. Is this common?*

A. A single umbilical artery, or a two-vessel cord, occurs in 0.5 to 1 percent of births in chromosomally normal babies and in 10 percent of chromosomally abnormal babies. In most normal babies, a two-vessel cord is the only abnormality present in the fetus.

Q. *Is my two-vessel baby at any risk during pregnancy or delivery?*

A. No. The placenta works fine. Your baby will get good nutrition and oxygen and grow normally. Your baby will tolerate labor and delivery as well as any other baby. All chromosomally normal babies with two vessels that look normal have normal kidneys.

Q. *Can my doctor see if the cord is wrapped around my baby's neck during the ultrasound?*

A. Yes, the cord can be seen wrapped around the baby's neck in a third-trimester ultrasound exam about one-third of the time.

Q. *What is the significance of the cord wrapped around my baby's neck?*

A. There is no increase in fetal growth restriction (FGR)—that is, low-birth-weight babies. A large study has shown that the stillborn rate, which was extremely low, was the same for babies with or without cords wrapped around their necks. The incidence of cesarean section due to nonreassuring heart rate patterns was not really increased.

Q. *What is a biophysical profile?*

A. This screening test employs the use of both the external fetal monitor and the ultrasound machine. First, a nonstress test is performed and is followed by an ultrasound exam. During the ultrasound, your doctor will look at the amount of amniotic fluid, fetal muscle tone, breathing movement, and limb or body movements. Each of the categories receives a score of 0 (abnormal) or 2 (normal). A low score may indicate the need for delivery, especially if the pregnancy is near term.

AMNIOCENTESIS

Q. *What is amniocentesis?*

A. Amniocentesis is a diagnostic test that involves the removal of amniotic fluid with a needle that goes through your abdomen and into your uterus.

Q. *How is it performed?*

A. First, an ultrasound is done to determine that there is an adequate amount of amniotic fluid to remove and an area free of placenta and baby where the needle can be inserted. Your abdomen is then cleaned, and a local anesthetic may or may not be injected into your skin at the site where the amniocentesis needle will be inserted. Then, with the help of the ultrasound, a long needle is guided into your uterus (avoiding the placenta and your fetus), and a small amount of amniotic fluid is removed.

Q. *Why is amniocentesis performed?*

A. This test can determine chromosomal disorders (for example, Down syndrome or Tay-Sachs disease), fetal lung maturity, neural tube defects, severity of Rh disease, or intrauterine infections. It is also used in paternity testing.

Q. *When is amniocentesis performed to detect genetic abnormalities?*

A. A genetic amniocentesis is usually performed between the 15th and 17th week of your pregnancy. An early amniocentesis can sometimes be performed at 13 weeks.

Q. *What are the complications of amniocentesis?*

A. The risk of complications is low, less than 0.25 percent. The major risk is miscarriage, which occurs in about 1 in 400 cases. You may also (rarely) experience temporary cramping, scant bleeding, or amniotic fluid leakage, which usually stop on their own and do not need treatment other than bed rest. Severe bleeding, infection, miscarriage, and death have occurred, but are extremely rare events. If you are Rh-negative, you should have an injection of Rh immune globulin after the procedure. With the use of ultrasound, the fetus, cord, and placenta are rarely stuck by the needle. If performed near term, rupture of membranes or the initiation of labor rarely occurs. As with any procedure, the benefits should outweigh the risks.

Q. *Why should I have a genetic amniocentesis?*

A. Have the test if you want to know if you have an affected child so you can decide on your plan of action—fetal surgery, education and preparation for a special-needs child, paternity information, pregnancy termination.

Q. *Why should I not have a genetic amniocentesis?*

A. Don't have the test if the risks of miscarriage are too high for you to tolerate or if you know that based on your moral, ethical, and religious principles, you would not terminate a pregnancy for any reason. Also, you may not feel the need to be mentally prepared for a special-needs child.

GROUP B STREPTOCOCCUS (GBS)

Q. *Why test for GBS?*

A. Group B streptococcus, or GBS, is a bacterium normally found in the intestines, bladder, and genital tract of up to 30 percent of healthy adult men and women. A pregnant woman who tests positive for GBS can pass the GBS to her baby during a vaginal delivery. The baby then has a 1 in 300 chance of becoming ill.

Q. *If I test positive for GBS, why don't I have symptoms of an infection?*

A. Most of the time, there are no symptoms and you are just colonized with the bacteria. An overgrowth of vaginal GBS can cause an infection causing a discharge and irritation. Asymptomatic, colonized pregnant women do not need to be treated until they go into labor.

Q. *Is GBS sexually transmitted?*

A. No. You can't transmit GBS through oral sex either. Strep throat is caused by group A streptococcus.

Q. *How is the GBS test performed?*

A. The GBS test is a simple and rapid test to perform. The doctor will place a cotton swab at the opening of your vagina and another at the opening of your rectum for culture. It is performed during your 35th to 37th week. The results will be ready in 2 days.

Q. *What kind of an infection can GBS cause in my baby?*

A. One in 200 babies may become infected and sick after a vaginal delivery. There are two types of infection—an early-onset and a late-onset infection. The early-onset infection will occur between 6 hours and 7 days from vaginal delivery. The most common infections are pneumonia, meningitis, and sepsis (blood infection), which on rare occasion can be fatal. The less common, late-onset infection occurs from a week to several months after vaginal delivery and may also result from an infection from someone with GBS who contacts your baby. The most common infection is meningitis.

Q. *If I test positive for GBS, can I be treated immediately to prevent an infection in my baby?*

A. Treatment with oral antibiotics before labor will only decrease the amount of GBS in your vagina temporarily. The bacteria grow very rapidly, and therefore, treatment before labor will not protect your baby from potential infection. Treatment is begun in the hospital when you are in labor. You will receive IV antibiotics. Penicillin is the treatment of choice. Another antibiotic will be administered if you are allergic to penicillin. Untreated babies have a 1 in 300 chance of becoming infected. Treated babies are twenty times less likely to become infected, with only 1 in 6,000 becoming ill.

Q. *Do I need to be treated for GBS if I am having a planned C-section?*

A. No.

Q. *Do I need to be tested for GBS if
I am having a planned C-section?*

A. Yes. You may go into labor before your planned C-section date. You may spontaneously rupture your membranes before your planned C-section date.

Q. *If my urine culture tested during
my first OB visit tested positive for GBS,
do I need to be tested in my third trimester?*

A. No, you are positive for GBS. You should be treated for the positive bladder infection now with oral antibiotics and treated during labor with IV antibiotics.

Q. *If I tested positive for GBS in a
previous pregnancy, should
I get tested during this pregnancy?*

A. You could, but I recommend just getting treatment during labor.

Q. *What happens if I go into labor
before I've had my GBS test?*

A. Women with an unknown GBS status who go into preterm labor, who prematurely break their water, or who have ruptured membranes for more than 18 hours should receive IV antibiotic treatment.

Q. *Will the antibiotic treatment
hurt my baby?*

A. No.

Q. *Do I have to have treatment of my positive GBS during labor?*

A. You can refuse treatment and play the odds. It is your choice.

TOXOPLASMOSIS

Q. *What is toxoplasmosis?*

A. This is an infection caused by a one-celled parasite called *Toxoplasma gondii.*

Q. *What are the symptoms of toxoplasmosis?*

A. Most of the time there are no symptoms upon contracting the infection. Symptoms, when they do occur, are nonspecific: fever, fatigue, and swollen lymph nodes.

Q. *How do I get a toxoplasmosis infection?*

A. You can contract this disease by coming into contact with infected cat feces, eating contaminated raw vegetables, fruits, or undercooked meats, and by gardening without gloves in contaminated soil. About 40 percent of pregnant women have had prior exposure to toxoplasmosis and are immune to subsequent exposure. About 1 in 8,000 babies per year in the United States are born with toxoplasmosis.

Q. *Is there a test I can take to find out if I have toxoplasmosis?*

A. Yes. It is a blood test that will tell you if you have a recent or past infection.

Q. *If I become infected with toxoplasmosis during my pregnancy, will my baby become infected?*

A. The risk of infection to the fetus depends on the stage of your pregnancy: 5 percent in the first trimester, 30 percent in the second trimester, 60 percent in the third trimester. Most congenital infections are mild or have no apparent effect, especially if contracted late in pregnancy, where almost 90 percent of babies appear to be normal. However, if infection occurs in the first trimester and the fetus becomes infected as well, up to 75 percent may develop severe problems, such as blindness, hydrocephalus, or mental retardation.

Q. *Can a strictly indoor cat transmit toxoplasmosis?*

A. No, not unless you feed your cat infected raw or undercooked meat.

ELECTRONIC FETAL MONITORING

Q. *What is external fetal monitoring?*

A. External fetal monitoring is performed by a machine that records the fetal heartbeat and your uterine contractions. An ultrasound device called a transducer, which uses sound waves (like the doptone instrument), picks up the fetal heart rate, and a pressure monitor placed on your abdomen detects uterine contractions. The machine then records this information on a moving strip of paper. The external fetal monitor is used to perform nonstress tests and contraction stress tests as part of the biophysical profile and to monitor your baby and contractions during labor.

Q. *What is internal fetal monitoring?*

A. There are two devices used for internal fetal monitoring: the scalp electrode and the internal pressure transducer. Both instruments require your cervix to be dilated enough for your doctor to place the devices inside your uterine cavity. Your amniotic sac must also be ruptured, either spontaneously or artificially by your doctor. The scalp electrode is a small, thin wire shaped like a corkscrew. It is attached very superficially to your baby's scalp for a more accurate recording of the heart rate. The internal pressure transducer is a thin water-filled tube that will accurately record the strength and duration of each uterine contraction. The catheter is placed through your dilated cervix around your baby's head and settles in between your baby's body and the inside wall of your uterus in your uterine cavity. The catheter is soft and pliable and will not injure your baby or uterus.

Q. *When is a fetal scalp electrode used?*

A. Scalp electrodes are not used routinely in labor. A scalp electrode may be employed if a good signal cannot be obtained using an external monitor, as is the case in an obese mom, in a pregnancy complicated with polyhydramnios (the baby has too much room in which to move away from the external transducer), or in a laboring mom who is moving around too much because of intense labor pains. A scalp electrode may also be used to more closely and accurately monitor the heart rate tracing if the fetal heart rate tracing is nonreassuring on the external fetal monitor.

Q. *When is the internal pressure transducer used?*

A. The internal pressure catheter is not used routinely during labor. Your doctor may choose to usee the catheter to more accurately monitor the strength of your uterine contractions if your labor progress has stopped and your cervix is not dilating, after placement of an epidural, or, in an obese mom, to monitor contractions not picked up by an external monitor. Some doctors use an internal pressure catheter when using Pitocin (oxytocin) for augmentation of labor. The internal pressure catheter may also be used for amnioinfusion (see Chapter 10).

Q. *Will my labor be monitored?*

A. This is a question that can only be answered by your doctor. It has become routine in most hospitals.

Q. *Can I move in bed while I am being monitored?*

A. Of course you can. If the external monitor is used, your nurse will readjust the instruments if need be; the internal monitors are not affected by movement.

Q. *Can the fetal monitor help me and my coach during labor?*

A. Yes. Your coach can see when a contraction is starting and inform you when the peak of a contraction is occurring. This may be a great help in modifying your relaxation and breathing techniques.

Q. *Can my baby get an electric shock*
from the internal scalp electrode?

A. No. Electric current does not pass along this line.

TESTS FOR FETAL WELL-BEING

Q. *What are the tests for fetal well-being?*

A. The nonstress test (NST), contraction stress test (CST), bio-physical profile (BPP), and fetal kick count are all tests for fetal well-being.

Q. *What are some indications for*
monitoring the health of my baby?

A. Here are some indications for fetal monitoring:

- Decreased fetal movement
- Low fetal kick count
- Postterm pregnancy
- Fetal growth restriction (small baby)
- Toxemia
- Maternal high blood pressure
- Maternal diabetes mellitus
- Oligohydramnios (too little fluid)

- Polyhydramnios (too much fluid)
- High AFP in a fetus without a neural tube defect
- Preterm rupture of the membranes at bed rest
- Multiple-birth pregnancy

FETAL KICK COUNT

Q. *What is the fetal kick count?*

A. This is a test that can be performed by you at home anytime after the 28th week of your pregnancy. There are two ways to perform this test. You can count how many times the baby moves in 1 hour during the same time of day or count how many movements occur in a 1- or 2-hour time slot during the same time every day.

Q. *Why count fetal movements?*

A. If you are worried about the health of your fetus, this is an inexpensive, simple, and accurate method to reassure yourself that your fetus is well. You are also taking the time to relax and bond with your baby.

Q. *When should I do the kick counts?*

A. Try to find the same time to count movements every day. Counting kicks after a meal is ideal. If you work, then do your count in the evening after dinner. If you are a stay-at-home mom, good luck.

Q. *How do I count fetal kicks?*

A. Relax, sit down or lie down, and place your hand on your belly. Kicking, punching, head turning, rolling, squirming, and hiccups all count as movements.

Q. *Is the fetus more active at night?*

A. Some babies are more active at night, and other babies aren't. The fetus has its own sleep-wake cycle. For example, near term, the fetus usually is active for about 35 minutes, then is inactive or sleeps for about 20 minutes. You probably notice the movements more often at night in bed because you are not distracted by normal daytime activities.

Q. *Is the fetus more active after I eat a meal?*

A. Yes, food and ice-cold drinks may stimulate your baby to move.

Q. *Sometimes I think that I can feel the baby's heartbeat. What is this rhythmic movement I am feeling?*

A. This rhythmic flutter is actually fetal hiccups! Fetal hiccups begin in the middle of the second trimester and become more frequent in the third trimester. We do not know what causes fetal hiccups or why they occur. The presence of fetal hiccups throughout your pregnancy has no significance to the health of your fetus. So if you notice your fetus hiccuping, have fun with it.

Q. *What can decrease fetal movements?*

A. The use of alcohol, cigarettes, sedatives, narcotics, or other medicines all may decrease the movement of your fetus.

Q. *What is a good fetal kick count?*

A. A good fetal kick count is ten movements within 2 hours or at least the same (or more) number of movements that your baby usually does in 1 hour.

Q. *I have been counting kick counts for 2 hours, and my baby has moved fewer than ten times. What should I do?*

A. Walk around for a few minutes, then lie down on your left side and try to count kicks again. You can also drink a glass of an ice-cold beverage and try again or eat a piece of candy or other sugar-rich food. If the ten-movement criterion is still not met in another 2 hours, call your doctor.

Q. *My baby passes the kick count test, but it is taking longer and longer to feel the movements. Is that okay?*

A. Near the end of your pregnancy, your baby has less room in which to kick and punch. Your baby should still be actively squirming and wiggling and stretching. If you have noticed a distinct trend in a slowing down of your baby's movements, call your doctor.

NONSTRESS TEST

Q. *What is a nonstress test (NST)?*

A. The nonstress test is a test of fetal well-being. The external fetal monitor is utilized for this test. The fetal heart rate will be recorded, and you will be asked to mark down when you feel your baby move. A healthy baby's heart rate will speed up with its own movements. A good, or reactive, test will demonstrate variability of the heart rate and accelerations of the heart rate during fetal movement. This test may be done in the office or hospital anytime after the 30th week. The test usually takes no more than 45 minutes to perform. The test may be performed at weekly or twice weekly intervals until delivery.

Q. *What happens if I have a nonreactive nonstress test?*

A. Sometimes your baby may not move during the nonstress test. Your baby may be sleeping. Your doctor or nurse may try to wake your baby up using a device that makes a noise. A glass of ice water or food may also stimulate your baby to wake up. If your baby still does not move and the nonstress test still remains nonreactive, your doctor may perform other tests or suggest delivery.

BIOPHYSICAL PROFILE (BPP)

Q. *What is the biophysical profile?*

A. The biophysical profile is a test that combines ultrasound measurements with a nonstress test. During the ultrasound exam, your doctor or perinatologist will look at the amount of amniotic fluid, muscle tone, breathing movements, and limb or body movements. The ultrasound exam can take about 30 minutes to complete. Each of these categories receives a score from 0 to 2. A low score may indicate the need to deliver your baby.

CHORIONIC VILLUS SAMPLING (CVS)

Q. *What is chorionic villus sampling (CVS)?*

A. CVS is a diagnostic test that will identify a baby with chromosomal abnormalities or certain identifiable genetic disorders. It is performed at 11 weeks.

Q. *Who might want CVS?*

A. The most common patient undergoing CVS is one who will be thirty-five or older by the time of her delivery; the test will determine if she is carrying a baby with Down syndrome. Other indications, as with amniocentesis, are parents with a child with trisomy 21 (Down syndrome) or both parents carriers of an autosomal recessive disorder (cystic fibrosis, Tay-Sachs disease) or carriers of a sex-linked disorder (hemophilia). A large nuchal translucency measurement or a positive early biochemical marker blood test for a trisomy may be followed up with CVS. CVS may also be performed for paternity testing if the father of the baby is in question.

Q. *Is anything done before I have CVS?*

A. You will have an ultrasound exam to confirm the length of your pregnancy. A cervical culture for gonorrhea and chlamydia will be taken. A vaginal culture will also be performed. Your blood type and Rh should be sent to the perinatologist, who may prescribe RhoGAM (an Rh immune globulin) if you have Rh negative blood and your partner has Rh positive blood. You will also attend a genetics counseling session.

Q. *How is CVS performed?*

A. Using ultrasound for guidance, a thin catheter (tube) is placed through the cervix and into the uterus. The catheter is moved next to the growing placenta, and gentle suction is used to remove a small sample of tissue. An adequate amount of tissue is obtained 98 percent of the time. This procedure is as uncomfortable as a pelvic exam with a speculum.

Sometimes this transcervical method cannot be used because of an obstruction to the cervical opening or vaginal infections. In these cases, a transabdominal route is taken. Once again under ultrasound guidance, a long, thin needle is passed through your skin just above your pubic bone and into your uterus to obtain placental tissue. Again, successful sampling is obtained 98 percent of the time. Discomfort is minimized by the use of a local anesthetic to your skin. Both methods are office procedures.

Q. *How long does it take to get the results of the CVS?*

A. Preliminary results of the direct cell analysis are ready in 24 to 96 hours. The final culture results take about 2 weeks.

Q. *How safe is CVS?*

A. The major complication of CVS is miscarriage. The risk of miscarriage appears to be about 1 in 200, as compared to a loss rate of 1 in 350 to 400 with amniocentesis. Other complications may be cramping, pain at the puncture site, and infection.

Q. *What are the advantages of CVS over amniocentesis?*

A. The major advantage is the timing of the procedure; it is performed in the first trimester. Therefore, if a lethal or severe problem is identified with your fetus, a termination of pregnancy, if desired, can be performed during the first trimester. The abortion performed during the first trimester is safer than that performed after amniocentesis in the second trimester. The results are 99 percent accurate. Some genetic diseases diagnosed by CVS may be expressed in your baby to varying degrees of severity not measured by this test.

Q. *Does CVS test for everything that amniocentesis tests for?*

A. No. CVS will only test for chromosome anomalies and some inherited abnormalities. CVS can not detect neural tube defects or structural abnormalities (malformations). At 15 weeks gestation, you will be advised to take an alpha-fetoprotein (AFP) blood test to detect a neural tube defect. A follow-up ultrasound at about 22 weeks is also done to check for nonchromosomal congenital anomalies.

Q. *Where is CVS performed?*

A. CVS is performed all over the United States. The procedure is done by a perinatologist who has been trained, proctored, and certified to perform CVS. Your doctor will refer you to a center close to your home.

FIRST-TRIMESTER SCREENING

Q. *What is the nuchal translucency (NT) screening test?*

A. Performed by a perinatologist, this is an ultrasound test performed between 11 and 14 weeks in women over the age of thirty-five. First a crown-rump length measurement to verify the age of your baby will be performed. Then a measurement will be taken of the clear or black space in the back of your baby's neck.

Q. *What do the results mean?*

A. The results, combined with your age, will give you a numerical risk for having a baby with Down syndrome. The larger the nuchal translucency, the greater the risk will be. A normal nuchal translucency is less than 3 millimeters.

Q. *What if the NT is greater than 3 to 4 millimeters?*

A. An NT greater than 3 to 4 millimeters is found in less than 1 percent of pregnancies scanned and is associated with a high risk of chromosomally abnormal babies or babies with a heart abnormality.

Q. *What should I do if my baby's NT is high?*

A. You can request a CVS, await the results of the first-trimester biochemical marker blood test and then make a decision about further studies, await the results of the AFP quad test, wait until 17 weeks and decide to (or not to) do an amniocentesis after the second-trimester ultrasound.

Q. *How accurate are the results from the NT screening test?*

A. NT testing alone has a 5 percent false positive rate and will detect 65 percent of Down syndrome babies. Combined screening of NT measurement and blood test for pregnancy-associated plasma protein-A (PAPP-A) and free beta-HCG (-HCG) increases the detection rate to 83 percent with a false positive rate of 5 percent. Integrated (NT, PAPP-A, and free beta-HCG and AFP quad) screen detection increases the detection rate for Down syndrome to 88 percent with a false positive rate of 1 percent.

Q. *Why should I do a first-trimester screening?*

A. If you are over the age of thirty-five, your doctor will discuss all the different genetic screening tests that are offered to you. These tests can give you a relatively accurate assessment of your baby's risk of a chromosomal or heart abnormality without subjecting you to the risk of miscarriage by performing CVS or amniocentesis. A negative result this early in your pregnancy will greatly reduce your anxiety about having a chromosomally or structurally abnormal baby.

CARRIER SCREENING FOR INDIVIDUALS OF EASTERN EUROPEAN JEWISH DESCENT

Q. *What screening tests are available for Eastern European Jewish descendants?*

A. Prenatal testing is available for several autosomal recessive disease conditions that are more prevalent in this group. The American College of Obstetricians and Gynecologists (ACOG) recommends testing for Tay-Sachs disease, Canavan disease, cystic fibrosis, and familial dysautonomia. Other carrier screening disorders that may be tested include mucolipidosis IV; Niemann-Pick disease, type A; Fanconi anemia, group C; Bloom syndrome; and Gaucher's disease.

Q. *What is Tay-Sachs disease?*

A. Tay-Sachs disease is a fatal hereditary disorder of children due to the deficiency of the enzyme hexosaminidase A. A child born with Tay-Sachs disease will appear healthy and normal at birth. When the baby is four to six months old, signs and symptoms of this progressively deteriorating disorder of the nervous system will appear. These are loss of motor skills, blindness, deafness, mental retardation, seizures, inability to swallow, and finally a comatose state and death (usually within five years).

Q. *What are my chances of being a carrier of the Tay-Sachs gene?*

A. It is now known that being of Jewish ancestry increases your risk of being a carrier of this recessive gene. The risk in the Jewish population is 1 in 27. There is also a greater risk if you are Cajun or French-Canadian. However, approximately 1 in 150 non-Jewish individuals have decreased hexosaminidase A activity consistent with a Tay-Sachs carrier status or mutation.

Q. *Is testing for Tay-Sachs disease and the other disorders necessary if there is no family history of this disorder?*

A. Yes. More than 95 percent of couples with Tay-Sachs offspring have no family history of this disease. Because the screening test for Tay-Sachs has only been available for less than thirty years, it is possible that your parents, aunts, and uncles were never tested for carrier status. The only way to really know if this recessive gene runs in your family is if family members were tested or if a relative was born with the disease.

Q. *Who should be screened for Tay-Sachs disease?*

A. All Jewish, half-Jewish, Cajun, and French-Canadian men and women should be screened. If the couple consists of a Jewish and non-Jewish partner, the Jewish mate should be screened first. If the result is positive for carrier status, the other partner should be screened.

Q. *What does it mean to be a Tay-Sachs disease carrier?*

A. A carrier of this recessive gene is perfectly normal and healthy. However, when two people who are carriers reproduce, they have a 25 percent chance, with each pregnancy, of having an offspring with Tay-Sachs disease. If only one parent is a carrier, the offspring may become a normal healthy carrier but cannot get the disease.

Q. *What options are open to couples who are Tay Sachs carriers or carriers of other autosomal recessive disorders?*

A. You can have a chorionic villus sampling (CVS) or amniocentesis at the appropriate times to detect whether you will have an affected child. Another option is to elect not to have children. Or you can have children by artificial insemination by a noncarrying donor, or you can adopt.

FRAGILE X SYNDROME

Q. *What is fragile X syndrome (FXS)?*

A. Fragile X syndrome is the most common cause of inherited mental retardation. Impairment can range from a mild learning disability to severe intellectual deficits. FXS is also the most common known cause of autism, found is about 5 percent of cases.

FXS is an inherited disorder caused by a gene mutation. Carriers of the gene mutation are usually not affected. The fragile X mutation (permutation) may be passed on through generations without expression of the syndrome. When the permutation expands to a full mutation through a female carrier, the male will have FXS and the female will be affected, but to a lesser degree. Since this is an X-linked inherited disorder, a male with FXS or the permutation can pass it to his daughters but not to his sons.

Q. *Is there prenatal testing for FXS?*

A. If you have a family history if FXS or think that you do, ask your doctor to send you to a genetics counselor before you become pregnant. The counselor will determine if you may be a carrier and send you for a blood test that will detect if you are a carrier; results are usually ready within a month. If you are a carrier, you can discuss your options with the genetics counselor. The counselor may recommend testing for FXS by CVS or amniocentesis once you are pregnant to see if the fetus has the FMR-1 gene and is affected.

Q. *I am pregnant and am going to have a CVS or amniocentesis to test for Down syndrome. Can I also test for the FMR-1 gene to see if my fetus has FXS?*

A. Yes. Talk to the genetics counselor and perinatologist, and it will be done. No extra tissue or fluid is required, so there is no added risk to either procedure.

Q. *What are the mental and behavioral characteristics of FXS?*

A. Boys may have a short attention span and are very active. Most males have an IQ less than 70. They may not begin to talk until age three. Thy may exhibit behavioral patterns similar to those seen in an autistic child, such as pulling away from touch, hand biting, and poor eye contact. They may ask the same questions repeatedly, even after hearing the answer. Girls with FXS tend to be shy. They have a short attention span. About 30 percent have significant learning disabilities. Both boys and girls are sensitive to

noise and don't like a change in routine. They have fragile person-
alities and may have frequent tantrums.

Q. *What do FXS boys and girls look like?*

A. The boys typically have a large head with a prominent forehead and big ears; they have a high palate and can be cross-eyed.
They also have flat feet. At puberty, their face becomes more elon-
gated and their testicles and scrotum become somewhat enlarged.
    The girls may have large ears, flat feet, and flexible fingers.

Q. *Do FXS kids have any positive attributes?*

A. Yes. Although initially shy, they have a good sense of humor,
can imitate well, and have great memories.

Q. *How can I support my FXS child?*

A. There are many resources available. There are numerous
speech, language, occupational, and physical therapy programs.
There are special education programs at your local schools. If your
child demonstrates seizure activity, obsessive-compulsive behavior, attention deficit behavior, and hyperactivity, there are physicians and medicines that can help. For parental support, there is
the National Fragile X Foundation at the website fragilex.org.

CHAPTER 8

Obstetrical Complications
of Pregnancy

MISCARRIAGE

Q. *What is a miscarriage?*

A. Miscarriage, or spontaneous abortion, is the termination of pregnancy on or before 20 weeks. Most miscarriages (at least 80 percent) occur in the first trimester, usually before the end of the 8th week.

At least 60 percent of miscarriages are due to a chromosomally abnormal embryo. In fact, 50 percent of miscarriages are due to a "blighted ovum," or pregnancies where the embryo has died and only the placenta develops. The other 10 percent consist of genetic problems such as Down syndrome. The abnormal genetic material may come from the egg or the sperm. Sometimes the fertilized egg does not divide and multiply properly. Rarely, a miscarriage is caused by improper implantation into the uterine lining.

Q. *What is a threatened miscarriage?*

A. You may experience a small amount of vaginal bleeding with or without uterine cramping. This spotting usually occurs at the time of your missed period, just when you discovered that you were pregnant using your home pregnancy test, and is probably caused by implantation of the baby into your uterus. Your cervix is closed on exam. Your doctor may advise rest, bed rest, and avoidance of sex. Although this advice is commonly given, there is no proof that the rest helps prevent a miscarriage, but lying down my decrease your amount of bleeding and the intensity of your cramping.

Q. *What is an inevitable miscarriage?*

A. This type of miscarriage usually occurs at the end of the first trimester. You may notice a clear watery vaginal discharge that becomes tinged with blood. A speculum exam will reveal a cervix that is dilated and effaced with or without ruptured membranes or an undilated cervix with ruptured membranes. In any event, the prognosis is extremely poor, and you will be advised to complete the miscarriage by dilation and curettage (D&C) or medical therapy.

Q. *What is an incomplete miscarriage?*

A. You will have intense abdominal and/or back pain with a moderate to heavy amount of vaginal bleeding. Your cervix is open, and tissue can be seen. An ultrasound will reveal a fetus or placental tissue in your uterus. Bring in any tissue that you may have passed to your doctor. A D&C will be advised.

Q. *What is a complete miscarriage?*

A. The bleeding and cramping you experienced completely emptied out your uterus. Bring in any tissue that you may have passed to your doctor. Your cervix is closed, and an ultrasound verifies that your uterus has no remaining pregnancy tissue.

Q. *What is a missed miscarriage?*

A. A missed miscarriage occurs when the fetus dies but you are unaware of it (most of the time). There is no vaginal bleeding. Most women will experience pregnancy symptoms because although the fetus has died, the placenta is still functioning and making pregnancy hormones. These women will be shocked to learn that the fetus has no heart motion on ultrasound. Other women may be suspicious that they have a missed miscarriage because their pregnancy symptoms have disappeared before the end of the first trimester. A missed miscarriage may continue for months before your uterus naturally expels its contents. This was the case years ago before the advent of the ultrasound machine, which enabled practitioners to make this diagnosis in a timelier manner. Treatment is expectant management (waiting for spontaneous miscarriage, which could take weeks), medical management, or D&C.

Q. *What is a blighted ovum?*

A. This is also called an *anembryonic* pregnancy because an embryo (early fetus) never forms. On ultrasound, all one sees is an amniotic sac and placenta. Many times the yolk sac is absent. Some pregnant women are surprised; others, especially if they have been pregnant before, are suspicious that their pregnancy is not normal because they have mild or no pregnancy symptoms. Treatment is expectant management, D&C, or medical management.

Q. *What are the risk factors for miscarriage?*

A. Smoking, moderate drinking (alcohol), illicit drug use, excessive intake of caffeine, malnutrition, exposure to high doses of radiation, exposure to toxic substances, severe infections or illness, severe maternal trauma, and advanced maternal age can increase your risk for a miscarriage.

Q. *If I have had a miscarriage, how common is another one with my next pregnancy?*

A. Since more than half of all miscarriages are due to an abnormal fetus, your risk is about the same as it is for your age-group. If you have had two miscarriages in a row, your chances of having another are about 25 percent. The risk does not increase after the second miscarriage. Having three miscarriages in a row is extremely rare. This condition is called recurrent miscarriage or recurrent pregnancy loss and occurs in only 1 percent of couples. Be aware, however, that an increase in your age does increase your chances of having a miscarriage.

Q. *What are some myths about the causes of miscarriage?*

A. None of the following factors can cause a miscarriage:

- Emotional stress—anxiety, fear, anger, or fright (there is no evidence that emotions can cause a miscarriage)
- Working long hours
- Standing long hours
- Working a night shift
- Moderate exercise
- Sex
- Surgery in the first trimester (laparotomies, laparoscopies,

and other major surgeries have been successfully performed without an increase in the miscarriage rate)

Q. *How can I prevent a miscarriage?*

A. Since over half of miscarriages are due to abnormal chromosomes, there is not much you can do to prevent them. In general,
try to be in the best health you can. Exercise, eat a nutritious diet,
take your prenatal vitamins (or at least 400 micrograms of folic
acid), do not smoke, and do not drink alcohol.

Q. *What are the warning signs of a miscarriage?*

A. A subtle sign is the loss of the symptoms of pregnancy before
the end of your first trimester. You don't feel tired, your breasts
aren't sore, and your nausea, if once present, has disappeared. Most
miscarriages occur 1 to 3 weeks after the death of the fetus.

Vaginal spotting or bleeding is the most dramatic warning
sign with or without cramping. But remember, this occurs in about
20 to 40 percent of all pregnancies, and at least 50 percent of these
pregnancies will be normal—no miscarriage. The bleeding may be
due to implantation of the embryo, broken blood vessels in the
cervix, or a bleeding cervical polyp. Cramping usually does not occur until you are actually having a miscarriage.

Q. *If I am experiencing vaginal bleeding in
the first trimester, how do I know if I am
having a miscarriage?*

A. You don't know. This condition is called a threatened abortion. A general rule of thumb is that if you still have symptoms of

pregnancy, you probably still have a good pregnancy. If you are having spotting, your doctor may ask you to stay in bed and refrain from sexual intercourse for 24 to 48 hours. If your bleeding is heavier, you may be asked to undergo a pelvic examination to assess the size of your uterus or an ultrasound examination to look for signs of fetal activity. Initially, the doctor will look at your cervix. If the cervix is dilated, you are having a miscarriage; if not, a pelvic exam will be done to measure the size of your uterus. A uterus smaller than indicated by the length of your pregnancy will lead to an ultrasound exam to find the cause of this discrepancy. The fetal heart may be seen pumping by 6 weeks.

If you are less than 6 weeks pregnant, a blood test called a quantitative (number value) beta-HCG (beta human chorionic gonadotropin) may be drawn every other day to assess the growth of the pregnancy. Beta-HCG is a hormone made by the placenta, and its value almost doubles every 2 days; therefore, a healthy early pregnancy can be detected by this test. The combination of ultrasound, pelvic exam, and quantitative beta-HCG can also be used to diagnose an ectopic pregnancy (discussed later in this chapter).

Q. *What happens to me if I do have a miscarriage?*

A. This depends on the age of your pregnancy. If the pregnancy is less than 7 weeks, you may have a complete miscarriage; if greater than 7 weeks, more often than not the miscarriage is incomplete, the cervix is dilated, bleeding is brisk, and there is still part of the placenta inside your uterus. You will need a D&C.

Q. *What is a D&C?*

A. D&C stands for dilation and curettage. If the cervix is closed, it must first be opened, or dilated, to allow an instrument into the uterine cavity. Curettage is cleaning out the uterus. A plastic suction device is used. General or local anesthesia may be used for the procedure. The procedure takes less than 10 minutes and can be done in the doctor's office or in the hospital on a same-day basis.

Q. *What can I do after the D&C?*

A. Physical recovery after a miscarriage and D&C occurs very quickly. Your only restrictions will be to avoid sexual intercourse and douching for a period of time as designated by your doctor. If your blood loss was not excessive, and it usually isn't, you may resume your normal daily activities the following day. Emotionally, however, you may not feel up to doing anything for a period of time. You will be grieving and will go through the process of mourning.

Q. *How long can I expect to have vaginal spotting?*

A. You may have scant vaginal bleeding for up to 2 weeks after a miscarriage. Some women will have no bleeding for a few days after the D&C, and then bleeding may occur. Others may have bleeding on and off for 2 weeks. As long as the bleeding is not heavy, all these conditions are a normal postoperative course. If you experience heavy bleeding, fever, or chills, call your doctor.

Q. *How soon can we try again to conceive?*

A. There is no harm in trying to conceive as soon as you want to after a miscarriage. Your body will quickly recover, and you will ovulate 2 to 4 weeks after your miscarriage. If you are emotionally ready, so is your reproductive system.

Q. *If I have Rh-negative blood, do I need Rh immune globulin?*

A. Yes, you should get an injection of RhoGAM within 72 hours of your miscarriage.

ABRUPTIO PLACENTA

Q. *What is abruptio placenta?*

A. Abruptio placenta is the premature separation of the placenta after the 20th week of pregnancy and before the baby has been delivered. This condition may be dangerous, because when the placenta detaches, the fetus loses some of its supply of blood and oxygen. Since the site where the placenta attaches is filled with blood vessels, detachment causes bleeding from this area in the uterus.

Q. *What are the signs of abruption?*

A. Heavy vaginal bleeding with severe abdominal pain with or without regular uterine contractions occurs with an advanced stage of placental detachment. The amount of bleeding and degree of pain is proportional to the amount of placental separation. In about 33 percent of cases, the detachment is small, and only a bit of spotting may be noticed.

Q. *How common is abruptio placenta?*

A. Placental abruption occurs in about 1 in 250 pregnancies. About 50 percent of these occur before the 36th week of pregnancy.

Q. *Who is at risk for getting an abruption?*

A. Abruption occurs more frequently in pregnancies complicated by chronic hypertension, toxemia, diabetes, twins, moms older than thirty-five, smokers, poor nutrition, and past history of abruption. Abdominal trauma causing an abruption is rare. Using cocaine in the third trimester may cause an abruption.

Q. *What happens if I have an abruption?*

A. This, of course, depends on the degree of placental detachment. If only a small area detaches, your bleeding will have been transient, and watchful waiting with decreased activity will be required. If a larger area detaches and bleeding and labor ensue, an early delivery will result. If bleeding is very heavy and signs of fetal distress are noted, an emergency cesarean section may be performed.

PLACENTA PREVIA

Q. *What is placenta previa?*

A. The placenta has implanted low in the uterus and has grown near or over the internal opening of the cervix. As you approach the end of your pregnancy, the lower segment of the uterus begins to thin out, and the cervix may begin to efface and dilate, causing part of the placenta to detach from this area and resulting in "painless vaginal bleeding," the cardinal sign of placenta previa.

Placental previa in the third trimester is rare. The incidence of placenta previa is 1 in 200 pregnancies (0.5 percent). It is more common in women who have already had children: only 10 percent occur in first full-term pregnancies. Women having more than four pregnancies have a 1 in 20 chance of having placenta previa with their next pregnancy.

Q. *What causes placenta previa?*

A. The cause of the low placental implantation is not known, but we do know some of the risk factors. As already stated, prior pregnancies increase the likelihood of placenta previa. The incidence is doubled in twin pregnancies, probably because of the increased size of the placenta. The incidence is tripled in a pregnancy following a cesarean section with a low transverse scar (D&C). Previous induced and spontaneous abortions and prior dilation and curettage also increase risk owing to scarring of the uterus. Cigarette smoking during pregnancy doubles your risk because of the effects of carbon monoxide. Women over the age of thirty-five may have double the risk.

Q. *If I experience painless vaginal bleeding, what should I do?*

A. Call your doctor immediately. The first episode of bleeding (there can be more than one) is usually sudden in onset, painless, and profuse. Your clothes will become soaked with bright red blood, and seeing this may cause you to faint. The blood loss, which may be only scant spotting or as much as a cup or two, rarely causes shock; death is extremely rare and your baby is fine.

Q. *If I have a placenta previa, when is the most common time for bleeding to occur?*

A. The first bleeding episode usually occurs around the 30th week of your pregnancy.

Q. *What will the doctor do?*

A. The doctor will meet you at his or her office or at the hospital (if the diagnosis was made during an earlier routine ultrasound exam), depending on the amount of blood loss, whether you are still bleeding, and the time of day. The first episode of bleeding, although copious, is usually short-lived. An ultrasound examination will be performed to confirm or rule out a placenta previa. Ultrasound is accurate in 97 percent of cases. If you do have a placenta previa, management will depend on the maturity of your fetus. Your doctor will probably try to delay birth of your baby until the 35th week.

Q. *If my pregnancy is less than 35 weeks, what will happen next?*

A. You will be hospitalized for about 3 days, confined to bed for 48 hours, and then allowed to walk to the bathroom on the 3rd day. You will have an IV, and blood tests will be performed to check for anemia and to type and cross-match your blood in case you require blood replacement. You will need a blood transfusion if you are very anemic. You will receive two injections of steroids 24 hours apart to speed up the lung maturity of your baby. You will be discharged to home on bed rest only if you have stopped bleeding, if you live near the hospital, and if someone is with you at all times who can bring you back to the hospital if bleeding recurs. The doctor may ask you to have a blood test every 72 hours for cross-matching, so if profuse bleeding does recur, blood is immediately available for transfusion. In at least 75 percent of cases of placenta previa, the pregnancy will continue to the 36th week.

Q. *What happens if the bleeding continues?*

A. You will be taken to the operating room, and you will have a cesarean section. If the bleeding is heavy and your vital signs are not stable, you will have general anesthesia. If you are stable, spinal anesthesia may be administered.

Q. *If my pregnancy is 35 weeks or more, how will the doctor deliver my baby?*

A. The doctor will perform a cesarean section. If done on an elective basis, you will have your choice of anesthesia.

Q. *An ultrasound examination performed at 18 weeks showed a placenta previa. Does that mean I will need a cesarean section?*

A. Probably not. It has been shown that the incidence of placenta previa is much greater in the first and second trimesters than at term. During your advancing pregnancy, the placenta "migrates" away from the lower portion of the uterus, so your chances of having a placenta previa at term are only 1 in 20, as is your risk of cesarean section for this problem.

PLACENTA ACCRETA

Q. *What is placenta accreta?*

A. Placenta accreta is an abnormal adherence of the placenta to the uterus. This is due to the growth of the placenta deep into the endometrium of the uterus. Normally, the placenta attaches only superficially to the endometrium, or lining of the uterus. Placenta accreta may be partial or complete and is the most common abnormal attachment, accounting for 80 percent of cases.

Q. *How common is placenta accreta?*

A. Not very common at all. The reported incidence is about 1 in every 2,500 deliveries.

Q. *What is the treatment for placenta accreta?*

A. If the diagnosis was made before your delivery, your doctor will schedule a cesarean section. Blood will be available for replacement if necessary. Management is much easier if delivery is by cesarean section. In this case, if the accreta is partial, bleeding may be minimized and the placenta may be removed and the uterus repaired. If the accreta is complete and/or blood loss has been great, hysterectomy is the only treatment alternative.

INCOMPETENT CERVIX

Q. *What is an incompetent cervix?*

A. An incompetent cervix is a cervix that painlessly dilates during the second trimester or early third trimester, causing premature rupture of the membranes. Classically, you will not experience uterine contractions until after your membranes rupture. Soon after, you will miscarry your fetus. Incompetent cervix is rare. The incidence varies from 1 in 150 to 1 in 2,000 pregnancies.

Q. *What causes an incompetent cervix?*

A. There is no real cause of an incompetent cervix, but we know that it occurs more frequently in women with a history of incompetent cervix in a prior pregnancy or a history of a deep loop electrical excision procedure (LEEP) used to treat dysplasia, a precancerous condition, multiple D&Cs, multiple abortions (especially second-trimester abortions), a congenitally malformed cervix, DES exposure as a fetus, extensive damage to the cervix after a difficult vaginal delivery, or placenta previa in a prior pregnancy.

Q. *How will I know if I have an*
incompetent cervix?

A. Unless you have a history of incompetent cervix in a prior pregnancy, you won't. If you have some of the other risk factors, your doctor may be vigilant and do serial pelvic exams or ultrasounds to check for signs of incompetent cervix in your present pregnancy.

Q. *What is the treatment for a pregnancy with*
a prior history of incompetent cervix?

A. The treatment for incompetent cervix is surgical. Your doctor will place a suture around your cervix. This is called a *McDonald cerclage.* It is performed between 12 and 14 weeks as an outpatient procedure. The success rate—meaning, you will not have a second- or early third-trimester delivery—is 90 percent.

Q. *What are the complications of
the cerclage procedure?*

A. Complications, such as infection or bleeding, are rare. Occasionally, the procedure will trigger preterm labor (PTL), which can be halted by tocolytic medications. The most common problem is a heavy, nonodorous, thick yellow vaginal discharge.

Q. *What are my restrictions throughout
the remainder of my pregnancy?*

A. After the procedure, you should plan on limiting your activities for a few days. Exercise and other strenuous activities should be curtailed. Sexual relations, although allowed, should probably be kept to a minimum until at least 35 weeks.

Q. *When is the cerclage removed?*

A. The cerclage is usually removed at 36 to 38 weeks gestation. It is removed in the labor and delivery area of the hospital because at least one-third of patients will go into labor immediately after the suture is removed.

Q. *What is an emergency cerclage?*

A. Very rarely, a patient will present to her doctor complaining of a profuse mucous discharge between 16 and 24 weeks. On pelvic exam, the cervix is found to be dilated and the amniotic sac, or "bag," is bulging at the cervical opening. An emergency cerclage can be attempted. The success is limited but worth a try. The alternative is bed rest.

PREGNANCY-INDUCED HYPERTENSION (PIH)

Q. *What is PIH?*

A. Pregnancy-induced hypertension (PIH), also called *toxemia* or *preeclampsia*, is a disorder that usually occurs in the third trimester. There is a sudden increase in your blood pressure to 140/90, with the appearance of protein in your urine. As your blood pressure gets higher, your weight gain increases from water retention, which causes edema, or swelling, in your hands, face, and legs. Most cases are mild. Nationwide, it occurs in about 5 to 8 percent of pregnancies. It is most common in patients who are pregnant for the first time.

Q. *What are the risk factors?*

A. Being pregnant for the first time is a risk factor, since 65 percent of preeclampsia cases occur in first-time mothers. It is even more common if the mother-to-be is under the age of seventeen or is thirty-five or older. Afro-Americans have a higher incidence of preeclampsia. PIH is three times as common with a twin pregnancy. It is also more common in women with obesity, lupus, antiphospholipid antibody syndrome, diabetes, chronic hypertension, or kidney disease. There seems to be a familial tendency toward the development of toxemia. You are more likely to have PIH if your mother or sister had PIH.

Q. *How can PIH be prevented?*

A. There is no way to prevent PIH. If you have risk factors, get them under control. If you are obese or diabetic, try to lose weight and start an exercise regimen before your pregnancy. Make sure your hypertension is treated with medicines that are safe to use during your pregnancy. During your pregnancy, eat well-balanced meals, exercise daily, and get enough rest a night.

Q. *What are the symptoms of mild PIH?*

A. You may not notice any symptoms. Many times mild PIH is found during your routine prenatal visit. Your doctor will note that you have high blood pressure, protein in your urine, and a modest amount of weight gain with edema.

Q. *What is the treatment for mild PIH?*

A. If you are near the end of your pregnancy and your cervix is ripe, the treatment is labor and delivery. If you develop PIH early in the third trimester, the treatment is modified bed rest throughout most of the day and a diet high in protein. You will be seen by the doctor twice a week and will undergo a nonstress test at least weekly. Delivery by induction will occur when your cervix is ripe, or, if the severity of the disease progresses, induction and/or cesarean section will be performed regardless of the state of your cervix.

Q. *What are the complications of PIH?*

A. The major complication of mild PIH for the mother is the progression to the severe form with the development of blood-clotting problems, liver dysfunction, seizures, and, very rarely, death. Severe PIH requires hospitalization to stabilize your condition.

Q. *Are there warning signs for severe PIH?*

A. Yes. Headache, blurred vision, swelling of hands and face, decrease in urination with very concentrated urine, and pain under the right side of your rib cage are all warning signs. Notify your doctor immediately if any of these symptoms occur. The criteria for severe PIH is blood pressure of 160/110 or higher.

Q. *Is PIH dangerous to my baby?*

A. PIH causes the placenta to work less effectively, thus providing less nourishment to the fetus. As a result, the fetus will not grow as well and will be born with a low birth weight. If you develop severe PIH in the early third trimester and require an early delivery, your baby will also have to contend with the complications of prematurity.

Q. *Are there any special precautions during labor?*

A. You will have an IV and receive internal fetal monitoring. You will receive magnesium sulfate, a drug that prevents convulsions, through your IV during labor and, if you have severe PIH, for 24 hours after delivery. Magnesium sulfate is safe for your baby. The side effects of this therapy to you may be unpleasant. You may feel uncomfortably drowsy and warm, you may have double vision, and your tongue will feel thick.

Q. *What happens after delivery?*

A. Delivery is the cure for PIH. Your blood pressure usually returns to normal, and the increased water weight begins to disappear within 48 hours.

Q. *If I developed PIH with my first pregnancy, will I have it again with my next pregnancy?*

A. Probably not. The recurrence of PIH in subsequent pregnancies is only about 10 to15 percent, but your doctor will be watching for it

Q. *What is HELLP syndrome?*

A. Women with severe PIH and liver damage have this syndrome:

H: Hemolysis, the destruction of your red blood cells, causing anemia
EL: Elevated liver enzymes due to damage to your liver
LP: Low platelets, which can causing blood-clotting
   problems

This syndrome is rare, only present in 20 percent of cases of severe preeclampsia. Stabilization and delivery is the cure.

SHOULDER DYSTOCIA

Q. *What is shoulder dystocia?*

A. Shoulder dystocia is a difficult delivery due to the size of the baby's shoulders. The baby's head delivers but the shoulders are stuck in the mother's pelvis.

Q. *How common is shoulder dystocia?*

A. Shoulder dystocia occurs in 1 in 250 to 350 deliveries. The in-cidence of shoulder dystocia is higher for infants weighing less than 9 pounds because there are so many more infants born that weigh less than 9 pounds.

Q. *Who is at risk for shoulder dystocia?*

A. Pregnancies at risk for shoulder dystocia are those complicated by diabetes, maternal obesity, a previous infant weighing 9 pounds or more, possibly a labor with a prolonged active phase, and a fetus with an estimated weight of more than 9 pounds. Apparently, 55 percent of cases of shoulder dystocia occur in diabetic moms with large babies. The other 45 percent of cases are unpredictable and unpreventable.

Q. *What are the possible complications*
of shoulder dystocia?

A. The main complication is a brachial plexus injury to your baby, which can occur in up to 40 percent of cases. Most of the time, this nerve injury is temporary, and less than 10 percent of cases persist after the first year of life. The other complications of shoulder dystocia include broken clavicle, broken arm, depressed infant (one that has poor muscle tone, delayed or slow neurological handicap due to lack of oxygen or breathing, and slow heartbeat), and—extremely rarely—death.

Q. *How should I have my next delivery*
if I had a shoulder dystocia with my first delivery?

A. The recurrence risk of shoulder dystocia can be as high as 16 percent in some studies, but the real risk of recurrence is not known because many doctors and moms will automatically choose to have a cesarean section. Discuss the possible recurrence risks with your doctor, and choose your preferred mode of delivery before you go into labor.

BREECH

Q. *How common is a breech presentation?*

A. At term, the incidence of breech presentation (baby's butt the first part to deliver) is about 3 percent; however, it is much more common early in your pregnancy. About 33 percent are breech (feet or foot the first part to deliver).

Q. *If I have a breech baby past 36 weeks, will it turn?*

A. From 37 weeks on, the chances of spontaneous turning is rare. However, if desired, you may ask your doctor about external cephalic version.

Q. *What is external cephalic version?*

A. This is the turning of the fetus from the breech to the vertex (head-down) position. It is performed in the hospital after an ultrasound exam to confirm fetal position and well-being. The attempt will not be performed if the umbilical cord is wrapped around the baby's neck or the placenta is not in a good position. This will eliminate about 50 percent of candidates. You may have an IV with terbutaline—a uterine muscle relaxant. The doctor, usually a perinatologist, will then turn your baby by the gentle pushing of your baby's head and butt. This may take up to 10 minutes and is only mildly uncomfortable. The success rate for turning is as high as 50 percent. The procedure is safe, with an extremely low incidence of complications.

Q. *Aren't there natural techniques to turn my baby?*

A. Many natural techniques have been proposed to turn your baby to a head-down position. The pelvic tilt, music, burning herbs, chiropractic maneuvers, and more have been used with purported success before 37 to 38 weeks.

Q. *If I don't want external cephalic version, how will my baby be delivered?*

A. Most doctors will perform a cesarean section. The chance of a negative outcome for your baby, both in terms of birth trauma and death, is higher with a vaginal delivery. This is because the largest part of the baby to deliver in a breech presentation is the head. The body may easily deliver through an incompletely dilated cervix. The baby's larger head may get stuck at the cervical opening, and this may cause a difficult birth even with the use of forceps, with trauma to both mother and baby. There are doctors who will perform a vaginal delivery in selected cases.

Rh DISEASE

Q. *What is the Rh factor?*

A. The Rh factor is a protein found on the outside of the red blood cells of all rhesus monkeys. It is also found on most human blood cells. If it is on your red blood cells, you are Rh-positive; if it is not found on your red blood cells, you have Rh-negative blood.

Q. *How do I know if I am Rh-positive or Rh-negative?*

A. Your Rh status is tested as part of your prenatal panel blood work.

Q. *How does the Rh factor cause a problem?*

A. The problem occurs if your are an Rh-negative woman and you come into contact with Rh-positive red blood cells. Since this is a foreign substance to your bloodstream, your immune system will make antibodies to attack it. During pregnancy, especially in the last trimester, some of the Rh-positive fetal red blood cells may cross the placenta and enter your bloodstream. When this occurs during your first pregnancy, you will become sensitized and form antibodies. Usually, not enough antibodies form to cause a problem. But this antibody response is now primed. During a second pregnancy, as soon as a small amount of Rh-positive fetal red blood cells enter your circulation, you start to make Rh antibodies again—and this time in larger amounts. These antibodies are small enough to pass through the placenta and enter the bloodstream of your fetus. Once there, the antibodies attack the Rh-positive red blood cells and cause them to burst. This is called *hemolysis*. The fetus becomes anemic and jaundiced. Jaundice is a yellow appearance of the skin due to the breakdown products of hemoglobin from the broken blood cells. This hemolytic anemia can become so serious that it can cause brain damage and death of the fetus.

Q. *How common is Rh-negative blood?*

A. About 15 percent of the population has Rh-negative blood.

Q. *How common is Rh incompatibility?*

A. About 13 percent of couples have significant Rh incompatibility, where the mom has Rh-negative blood and the father has Rh-positive blood. If the mother has Rh-positive blood, it does not matter if the father has Rh-positive or Rh-negative blood.

Q. *Are there other ways for*
Rh sensitization to occur?

A. Yes, if incompatibility exists, Rh sensitization may occur after a miscarriage, induced abortion, subchorionic hemorrhage, ectopic (tubal) pregnancy, CVS, amniocentesis, vaginal delivery, or cesarean section.

Q. *How are Rh sensitization and hemolytic*
disease of the newborn prevented?

A. Rh hemolytic disease of your baby can be prevented by a vaccine of Rh immune globulin. The vaccine contains antibodies that will bind to any fetal red blood cell present in your circulation and therefore prevent your immune system from becoming stimulated to form antibodies of its own. It basically blocks this allergic reaction. These antibodies last only three months in your bloodstream, so repeated injections may be given.

Q. *When should I receive Rh immune globulin?*

A. It has been shown that receiving Rh immune globulin injection at 28 weeks and within 72 hours after delivery will prevent sensitization in 99.2 percent of Rh-negative mothers. The vaccine should also be administered after a miscarriage, ectopic pregnancy, CVS, and amniocentesis.

Q. *If I have a positive Rh titer, can I still receive the Rh immune globulin?*

A. No. This means that you are already sensitized; you are producing Rh antibodies.

Q. *If I have Rh-negative blood and I am going to have a postpartum sterilization, do I still have to receive the Rh immune globulin vaccine?*

A. Yes. You may decide to have your sterilization reversed, the procedure may fail to prevent another pregnancy, or, if you need a blood transfusion in the future, the presence of Rh antibodies interferes with cross-matching your blood.

ECTOPIC PREGNANCY

Q. *What is an ectopic pregnancy?*

A. An ectopic pregnancy is a pregnancy that grows outside of your uterus. The most common site for an ectopic pregnancy is in the fallopian tube (tubal pregnancy).

Q. *How common are ectopic pregnancies?*

A. Ectopic pregnancies occur in 1 in every 63 pregnancies. This is a threefold increase in cases since the early 1980s. This increase is thought to be due to an increase in the incidence of salpingitis (infection of the fallopian tubes) and improved methods of diagnosis and reporting.

Q. *Who is at risk for having an ectopic pregnancy?*

A. Any woman who has a partial blockage of the fertilized egg's passage down the fallopian tube is at risk. A past history of a tubal infection with gonorrhea or chlamydia increases a woman's risk, as does past surgery on the tube to correct an infertility problem. Women who become pregnant after tubal sterilization, who have had a previous ectopic pregnancy, or who are on the minipill or have an IUD are at increased risk.

Q. *What are the symptoms of an ectopic pregnancy?*

A. Most women miss their menstrual period and then complain of vaginal bleeding or spotting about 2 weeks later. About half also complain of pain in their lower abdomen, usually on one side. About 1 in 5 women have shoulder pain as well. Light-headedness or fainting occurs in 33 percent of the cases. Most of these symptoms occur within 6 to 8 weeks after the last normal menstrual period.

Q. *How does the doctor diagnose
an ectopic pregnancy?*

A. The doctor will be alert for signs of an ectopic pregnancy in a patient with a previous history of an ectopic pregnancy or with a high risk for having an ectopic pregnancy. This will ensure an early diagnosis and possibly a medical versus a surgical treatment. Your doctor may follow your pregnancy with serial beta-HCG (beta human chorionic gonadotropin) blood tests every 2 to 3 days during your early pregnancy until the blood levels are in the range where an intrauterine pregnancy may be detected by a vaginal probe ultrasound.

If you do not have a history of ectopic pregnancy, then the findings of a positive pregnancy test, ectopic pregnancy symptoms, a uterus smaller than expected for your stage of pregnancy, and a mass on the side of the pain will strongly suggest an ectopic pregnancy. A vaginal probe ultrasound at this point should help confirm the diagnosis.

Q. *Why is an ectopic pregnancy dangerous?*

A. The pregnancy will expand the tube and then rupture it, causing internal bleeding. If the diagnosis is delayed, massive blood loss, shock, or (rarely) death may result.

Q. *What is the treatment for an
ectopic pregnancy?*

A. Methotrexate is now the preferred method of treatment for ectopic pregnancies in selected early cases. Methotrexate stops the fast-dividing cells of the pregnancy from dividing and allows the tube to absorb the tissue. The success of this therapy has been quite good, as all the criteria for treatment are met. Methotrexate is given as two intramuscular injections in your buttocks. Your doctor will follow your beta-HCG until it is zero.

If the ectopic pregnancy has ruptured your tube or is causing you pain from the size of the pregnancy tissue and blood in your tube, you will require surgery. Your doctor will perform a laparoscopy under general anesthesia to remove the ectopic pregnancy with or without removing the tube, depending on the damage to the tube. A pregnancy in the tube will never grow for 40 weeks, nor can it be transferred into your uterus. The surgical removal of the ectopic pregnancy can usually be performed as an outpatient procedure using a laparoscope. If future pregnancies are desirable and the fallopian tube has not ruptured, the tube may be opened and the pregnancy removed without removing your tube. If the tube has ruptured or future childbearing is not desired, the tube may be removed through a laparoscopic procedure as well.

Q. What is laparoscopy?

A. Laparoscopy is a minor outpatient surgical procedure, usually performed under general anesthesia. After anesthesia has been employed, a needle is placed through your belly button and carbon dioxide gas is used to distend your abdomen. The laparoscope is then placed through the incision. The laparoscope is a small telescope attached to a video camera that enables your doctor to view your abdominal and pelvic organs on a video screen. Other very small incisions on your abdomen are used to place surgical instruments through to perform the removal of the pregnancy.

Q. *If I have had an ectopic pregnancy,*
what are my chances of having another one?

A. A repeat ectopic pregnancy may occur in 10 to 20 percent of subsequent pregnancies.

Q. *What are my chances of conceiving*
after an ectopic pregnancy?

A. A new study has shown that the answer to this question depends on the patient's previous obstetrical history. If the patient had no problem conceiving before her ectopic pregnancy, she will be successful again in the future. If she had a history of infertility, her chances of conceiving again will be decreased by as much as 50 percent.

PREMATURE RUPTURE OF MEMBRANES

Q. *What is premature rupture of*
membranes (PROM)?

A. This is a spontaneous break in the amniotic sac before the beginning of labor. There will be leakage of amniotic fluid from your vagina. The initial amount of fluid may be a cup or more or just a few drops of clear, yellow, or greenish fluid. If your water has broken, you will know because the leaking is continuous or recurrent.

Q. *What should I do if my membranes rupture?*

A. Call your doctor. You will be asked to go to the office or the hospital. If you are near term, there are usually no problems. Labor begins within 24 hours in up to 90 percent of patients. The problem occurs when the membranes rupture in a preterm pregnancy. This may occur in about 3 percent of pregnancies and is the cause of premature birth in 30 percent of cases. Preterm PROM in pregnancies less than 28 weeks occurs in less than 1 percent of pregnancies. If preterm PROM occurs between 28 and 34 weeks of pregnancy, about 50 percent of women will go into labor within 48 hours and 90 percent will be in labor after 1 week. If you experience preterm PROM before 32 weeks, you will stay in the hospital at bed rest. You will be given steroids to help mature your baby's lungs. Antibiotics will be administered to prevent infection. You will be allowed to deliver in 48 hours if labor is spontaneous, or you will be induced at 34 weeks. If preterm PROM occurs at 34 weeks, most doctors will allow you to go into labor or will induce labor.

FETAL GROWTH RESTRICTION (FGR)

Q. *How can I tell if my pregnancy*
is growing normally?

A. Your doctor will assess the growth of your baby by measuring your fundal height with a tape measure after 20 weeks. The fundal height measurement is taken from the top of your uterus, the fundus, to your pubic bone. The measurement in centimeters should equal the weeks of your pregnancy plus or minus 2 centimeters.

Q. *What is fetal growth restriction (FGR)?*

A. FGR is usually defined as a fetal weight that is less than 10 percent for gestational age. The fetus is not getting enough nutrition and has asymmetric growth—the head and brain grow normally but the abdomen does not.

Q. *How common is it?*

A. It may affect up to 5 percent of pregnancies in the general population.

Q. *How is FGR diagnosed?*

A. The routine fundal height exam will screen and detect most cases of FGR. Sometimes this method will not detect FGR in a mom who may be small in stature or an obese mom with extra fat in her tummy. An ultrasound exam will calculate the weight of your baby and make the diagnosis.

Q. *What are the risks for FGR?*

A. Risk factors include:

- Small mothers weighing less than 100 pounds
- Poor maternal weight gain due to poor nutrition
- Hypertension before pregnancy
- Preeclampsia
- Women living at very high altitudes
- Severe maternal anemia
- Smoking
- Heroin use
- Cocaine use
- Methamphetamine use
- Alcohol abuse
- Twins, triplets, quadruplets

- History of a previous FGR
- Chronic fetal infections—rubella, cytomegalovirus
- Postterm pregnancy—20 percent of babies
- Placental abnormalities
- Vessel umbilical cord
- Congenital anomalies

Q. *Is FGR dangerous to my baby?*

A. If the growth restriction is not severe, there is not much danger. But as the weight decreases below the 10th percentile, the risk of stillbirth increases.

Q. *How does the doctor confirm the diagnosis of FGR?*

A. Serial ultrasounds are performed at 2- to 4-week intervals. The doctor will measure the growth of the head, abdomen, and femur and will check for an adequate amount of amniotic fluid to confirm the diagnosis.

Q. *If my fetus has FGR and I am close to term, what will happen?*

A. FGR stresses the fetus, which usually speeds up lung maturity. Since the fetus is in an unfavorable environment, your doctor will elect to deliver your baby. Either induction of labor, if your cervix is ripe and the fetus responds well to the contractions of early labor, or a cesarean section will be performed.

Q. *What will happen if I am far from term with FGR?*

A. If a known cause (smoking, drinking, excessive physical exercise, or drug use) can be reversed, complete bed rest and monitoring of fetal well-being (nonstress test, contraction stimulation test, or biophysical profile) may be employed to gain days or weeks of intrauterine life. If the growth is minimal or the baby actually loses weight or if FGR is accompanied by oligohydramnios, delivery early in the third trimester may be anticipated. Your baby will grow better outside your uterus.

Q. *What are the possible complications of FGR?*

A. Your baby may have to be delivered prematurely, with the possible complication of respiratory distress syndrome of the newborn because of immature lungs. If the fetus undergoes distress during labor, the baby could be born without enough oxygen. Your chances of having a primary cesarean section and emergency cesarean section are greatly increased. The presence of meconium and meconium aspiration may occur. There is also an increased incidence of stillbirths.

Q. *Are there any problems with these babies later in life?*

A. In almost all cases of asymmetrical FGR, there is no long-term neurological or intellectual compromise.

Q. *What is oligohydramnios?*

A. There is a certain normal amount of amniotic fluid in your uterus. Too little amniotic fluid is called *oligohydramnios*. This problem most commonly occurs in the third trimester.

Q. *What causes oligohydramnios?*

A. The most common cause is a problem with the placenta; the placenta does not produce enough amniotic fluid. Certain conditions are complicated by oligohydramnios, including chronic hypertension, PIH, diabetes, and FGR. Pregnancies past 41 weeks are complicated by oligohydramnios at least 12 percent of the time.

Q. *How common is oligohydramnios?*

A. Very low levels of amniotic fluid occur in less than 5 percent of pregnancies.

Q. *How do I know if I have oligohydramnios?*

A. Your doctor will be suspicious if you have a predisposing factor. If your fundal height measurement is too small, oligohydramnios will be suspected and an ultrasound will be performed. The ultrasound will confirm the diagnosis.

Q. *What are the risks of oligohydramnios?*

A. The main risk is FGR. Stillbirths rarely occur. Labor problems due to umbilical cord compression with uterine contractions may lead to low oxygen to your baby, necessitating a cesarean section.

Q. *What is the treatment for oligohydramnios?*

A. The treatment depends on the age of your pregnancy. If you are not close to term, you will be placed on modified rest and instructed to drink at least eight glasses of fluid a day. Your diet should be reviewed and modified if your proteins and calories per day are inadequate. You will be monitored closely with a combination of ultrasounds, BPPs, and NSTs. If your pregnancy is close to term, the treatment of choice is delivery. If you have oligohydramnios during labor and an intrauterine catheter can be placed, an amnioinfusion will be performed to free the cord from compression during contractions.

Q. *What is polyhydramnios?*

A. Polyhydramnios is too much amniotic fluid. This condition usually occurs in the third trimester. It is not very common and occurs in less than 1 percent of pregnancies. The cause is unknown 65 percent of the time. The most common known cause is gestational diabetes.

Q. *How is the diagnosis made?*

A. You usually make the diagnosis yourself. You will notice a large increase in the size of your uterus. The fundal height measurement and ultrasound findings will confirm the diagnosis.

Q. *What are the risks of polyhydramnios?*

A. Preterm labor, premature rupture of membranes, placental abruption, stillbirth, and cesarean section are all potential events with polyhydramnios.

Q. *What is the treatment for polyhydramnios?*

A. You will be monitored closely with serial ultrasounds and BPP. If you are not close to your due date and you are uncomfortable, excess fluid may be removed by amniocentesis. This amnioreduction of fluid is temporary; the fluid will build back up. If you are near term, you will have your baby.

PRETERM LABOR (PTL)

Q. *What is preterm labor?*

A. Preterm labor is labor that occurs after the 20th week but before the 37th week of pregnancy. Up to 10 percent of pregnancies may end prematurely. The cause in more than 50 percent of the cases is unknown. The most common known cause is preterm premature rupture of membranes from unknown causes. We do know many of the risk factors for preterm labor.

Q. *What are the risk factors for preterm labor?*

A. Risk factors include the following:

- A previous history of preterm labor
- Family history of preterm labor
- Working a night shift (midnight to 8 a.m.)
- Premature rupture of the membranes
- A multiple pregnancy (twins, triplets, quadruplets)
- Congenital anomalies of the fetus
- Congenital anomalies of the uterus

- DES daughter (mother took diethylstilbestrol during her pregnancy)
- Prior uterine surgery (not a cesarean section)
- Incompetent cervix
- Abnormally large amount of amniotic fluid (polyhydramnios)
- Two or more second-trimester miscarriages or abortions
- Serious maternal diseases
- Poor nutrition
- Cigarette smoking
- Illicit drug use
- No prenatal care
- Age under eighteen

Q. *How do I know if I am in preterm labor?*

A. Many times you don't know. The difference between false labor and real labor is often difficult to establish, so call your doctor if you are unsure. There are some warning signs for preterm labor, but these signs may also be part of a normal, healthy pregnancy.

Q. *What are the warning signs of preterm labor?*

A. The most important warning sign is uterine contractions. The uterus is mainly composed of interlacing fibers of muscles. A uterine contraction is the tightening of the muscles of the uterus. During a contraction, you can feel your uterus become hard, and it will be difficult to indent with your fingertips. These contractions do not necessarily have to be painful. Preterm labor contractions do not have to be painful either, but these contractions definitely have a pattern to them. The entire uterus will become hard, and the contractions will last from 60 to 90 seconds and recur at least every 10 minutes. The contractions do not disappear with a change in position and become stronger in intensity with time. In addition to uterine contractions, there are several additional signs of preterm labor:

- A dull lower backache that may be rhythmic and constant and not relieved by a change in your position
- An increased feeling of pelvic pressure that feels like a fullness in the pelvic area
- Gas pains with or without diarrhea
- An increase in your vaginal discharge, which may become more mucous and watery or pink and blood tinged

Q. *How does my doctor know if I am in preterm labor?*

A. Sometimes, especially in very early preterm labor, the diagnosis is not always readily apparent. You will have a pelvic (speculum) exam. If your cervix has not effaced and is not dilated, it is possible that you are in early preterm labor or you are having strong Braxton Hicks contractions. A cotton swab will be placed under the cervix, and this specimen will be analyzed for the presence of fetal fibronectin. The test results are usually available in less than 4 hours. The absence of fetal fibronectin is reassuring in this scenario. The contractions, although intense for you, were only strong Braxton Hicks contractions. While waiting for this result, your doctor may give you a dose of terbutaline, which stops or greatly slows down the frequency and intensity of your uterine contractions. No other treatment will be necessary. If, however, your cervix has effaced and dilated in the presence of uterine contractions, the diagnosis of preterm labor will be made.

Q. *Can preterm labor be stopped?*

A. Yes, in many cases it can. The question of whether to stop labor is sometimes controversial and may depend on the reason for labor and the weight and age of your fetus. Doctors debate the gestational age limits for initiating tocolytic therapy. The latest age to try to stop labor is 34 weeks (The earliest age to allow labor is 34 weeks). This means that if you are in preterm labor at this point in your pregnancy, you will be allowed to go into labor and have your baby if initial therapy fails. Babies born at 34 weeks have an excellent chance for both survival and normal development but may have to spend a week in the hospital.

Initial therapy consists of complete bed rest and hydration with intravenous fluids. This therapy may be successful in almost 50 percent of cases of preterm labor. Terbutaline injections or magnesium sulfate (depending on physician's preference) administered through the IV will be used next, if needed. The medications will be continued for at least 24 hours after contractions have stopped. Success with these drugs may approach 70 percent.

A major factor for stopping labor depends on the state of effacement and dilation of the cervix at the onset of therapy. So if you think you are in preterm labor, don't hesitate to call your doctor or go to labor and delivery at your hospital.

Q. *What are the side effects of terbutaline?*

A. The side effects of this tocolytic are usually only experienced for the first day or two of therapy. Occasionally, the effects can be very uncomfortable. Your side effects may include:

- Increased heart rate
- Retention of fluid in the lungs, causing chest pains and shortness of breath
- Nausea, vomiting, or constipation
- Light-headedness
- Headaches
- Difficulty sleeping or jitteriness
- Fluctuating blood sugar levels

Q. *Are there any harmful effects of terbutaline on my baby?*

A. There is no increased incidence of birth defects or developmental problems from these medications. If your baby is born within 24 hours of therapy, his or her glucose level will be monitored for a low level. Treatment is feedings with a sugar solution.

Q. *What are the side effects of magnesium sulfate therapy?*

A. As with the other class of tocolytics, the side effects will usually last only 1 or 2 days. Initially, you may feel feverish, your tongue may feel thick, and you may experience headaches, double vision, nausea, and constipation. You my feel very drowsy and drift in and out of sleep owing to a somewhat unpleasant sedative effect.

Q. *Are there any effects of magnesium sulfate therapy on my baby?*

A. There is no increased incidence of birth defects or developmental problems associated with magnesium sulfate therapy. If your baby is born soon after a failed treatment with a relatively high therapeutic dose of magnesium sulfate still in your system, your baby's muscle tone may be decreased for the first hour or two of life.

Q. *What happens to me after my preterm labor has been stopped with IV therapy?*

A. There are three possible treatment scenarios for the continuation of treatment after labor has successfully been stopped. Treatment depends on many factors and physician practice. You may remain in the hospital for bed rest under observation for an additional day or two, taking oral doses of terbutaline or magnesium. Your doctor may order a subcutaneous pump that will administer doses of terbutaline through a needle placed in the fat layer under the skin continuously or at intervals determined by your doctor. You will also have the ability to give yourself additional doses of medications if your uterus becomes irritable or crampy or if you experience contractions.

Q. *If my baby is born prematurely, will he or she survive?*

A. Every year there are greater advances in the field of neonatal medicine, and the survival rate for premature infants is becoming better and better. Newborns born between 26 and 28 weeks of pregnancy have a good chance for survival but may have a 25 percent chance of having some type of long-term problem related to prematurity. Babies born after 30 weeks have an excellent survival rate and usually do not have long-term problems. But these statistics will get even better in the years to come. There have even been newborn survivors at 24 weeks.

Q. *How long will my premature
baby stay in the hospital?*

A. A good estimate is that most preterm infants remain in the hospital until their original due date. For example, if you delivered prematurely at 30 weeks gestation, your baby will be in the hospital for 8 to10 weeks.

Q. *I have a past history of preterm labor
(PTL) or preterm PROM. What can I do?*

A. If your history is consistent with delivering a preterm baby before 34 weeks, you may be a candidate for weekly injections of 17-hydroxyprogesterone starting at 16 weeks. This may prolong your next birth to 36 weeks or longer. This regimen is not harmful to your baby and may help by decreasing prematurity and its long-term complications.

Q. *How much does it cost to keep a baby
in a neonatal intensive care unit (NICU)?*

A. The average cost is between $1,000 and $2,000 per day. Check with your insurance company for coverage. Social services at the hospital will help you.

POSTTERM PREGNANCY

Q. *What is a postterm pregnancy?*

A. A postterm pregnancy is one that lasts more than 42 weeks, or 294 days, from the first day of the last menstrual period (LMP).

This definition assumes that the length of the previous menstrual cycles was 28 days. The average length of pregnancy lasts 40 weeks, or 280 days. About 85 percent of babies are born between 38 and 42 weeks. Only 5 percent of babies are born on their due date.

Q. *How common are postterm pregnancies?*

A. About 7 to 10 percent of all pregnancies last until 42 weeks, and 3 percent last more than 43 weeks.

Q. *What causes postterm pregnancies.?*

A. There are many theories, but we don't know the exact cause. The most common reason for a postterm pregnancy is error or guessing of dates of the LMP. If early ultrasound were used routinely, the incidence of postterm pregnancy would probably decrease from 10 percent to 3 percent.

Q. *If my first pregnancy was postterm,*
will this pregnancy be postterm, too?

A. If your first pregnancy was postterm, you have a 50 percent chance that your second pregnancy will go to 42 weeks.

Q. *What are the effects on my baby*
if it is postterm?

A. Most babies do well even if the pregnancy goes past 42 weeks, but there are potential problems. The perinatal death rate (stillbirths plus early neonatal deaths) doubles when waiting from 40 weeks to 42 weeks to deliver, from 2 or 3 per 1,000 to 4 to 7 per 1,000.

In about 20 percent of these pregnancies, the placenta will not supply enough nutrients to the fetus. Weight loss, decreased amniotic fluid, thin, fragile umbilical cords, fetal inability to tolerate labor, and increased presence of meconium and meconium aspiration may result. In another 20 percent of these pregnancies, the fetus will continue to grow to at least 9 pounds, with 3 percent of these babies weighing 10 pounds. These increased birth weights increase the incidence of cesarean section due to cephalopelvic disproportion (the head is too big to make it through the birth canal).

Meconium in the amniotic fluid occurs more commonly, in 27 to 43 percent of postterm pregnancies. At 40 weeks, the incidence of meconium-stained fluid is about 15 percent. Meconium may be a warning sign that the pregnancy is being compromised, especially if it is thick and there is little amniotic fluid. Careful internal fetal monitoring during labor will point out any potential signs of fetal distress.

Q. *What are my risks if I have a postterm pregnancy?*

A. Emotionally, you may be very anxious waiting an additional week or two past your due date to go into labor. As your baby grows larger, you can become more physically uncomfortable as well. If your baby does become heavier, your chance of having an abnormal labor doubles, the risk of severe vaginal tears is increased by 30 percent, and the chance of having a cesarean section because of a large baby or one with FGR is doubled.

Q. *What will my doctor do if my pregnancy is postterm?*

A. Your doctor will monitor the health of your fetus by using nonstress tests, contraction stress tests, and/or biophysical profile. If your pregnancy date is accurate and your cervix is ripe, induction of labor will be performed between your 40th and 41st week. If your cervix is not ripe, preinduction with a cervical ripening agent will be offered. Elective induction at 41 weeks results in lower incidence of cesarean sections, a lower perinatal death rate, and an overall better outcome for the babies induced rather than waiting to 42 week or longer. If there is any concern for the health of your baby, delivery by induction of labor or cesarean section will be performed.

TWINS

Q. *How common are twin pregnancies?*

A. In the United States, twins occur naturally in 1 out of every 93 deliveries. There are two types of twins: identical and fraternal twins. Identical twins come from one fertilized egg that splits early in the pregnancy. Fraternal twins come from two separate fertilized eggs. Fraternal twins are more common, constituting about 70 percent of twins born.

Q. *Are some women more likely to have twins?*

A. Fraternal twins are more common if you are a twin or your mother was a twin. Your husband's family history has no influence on the incidence of twins. Twins are also more common with the increasing age and number of pregnancies of the mother. Twins are more common in African-Americans (1 in 79). Twin pregnancies have become much more common since the popularity of fertility drugs and in vitro fertilization, increasing the multiple-birth rate to 1 in 33. Identical twins don't seem to be influenced by any factors and are constant throughout the world, with a birthrate of 1 in 250 births.

Q. *How do I know if I have twins?*

A. There are some clues. You may feel more nausea than a prior pregnancy or you may put on weight more quickly than expected. The rapid growth of the uterus after the first trimester may be felt by you or your doctor.

Q. *How will my doctor make the diagnosis of my twin pregnancy?*

A. An ultrasound will confirm the twin pregnancy in the first or second trimester, whenever your first ultrasound exam is performed.

Q. *What is the mean duration of a twin pregnancy?*

A. The mean duration is 37 weeks.

Q. *Is having twins considered a high-risk pregnancy?*

A. Yes. Having twins is considered a high-risk pregnancy. Fifty percent of twins will be born before 36 weeks. There is a 25 percent chance that your twins will be born premature, requiring that they be cared for in the NICU.

Q. *Is there a test to detect an increased risk of preterm labor?*

A. Yes. Cervical length measurement using transvaginal ultrasound in the second trimester can assess your risk for PTL. The length, along with presence or absence of funneling, may be used periodically throughout your pregnancy.

Q. *Besides prematurity, are there any other potential problems facing me and my babies?*

A. Major and minor malformations are twice as common with twins, being 2 percent and 4 percent, respectively. There is also a greater chance of morbidity and death of one baby during delivery, the rate being three times as common as with a single-child pregnancy. Preeclampsia occurs twice as often. This is due to the crowding of the second placenta by the first placenta. FGR of the second baby, or baby B, is always a concern and many times a reason for early delivery at 34 to 36 weeks. Anemia, bladder infections, FGR, abruption, and placenta previa are all more common than with single-baby pregnancies. By the 28th week, your uterus will be the size of a term pregnancy and will only grow larger. This means more frequent and more severe heartburn, back pain, joint pain, constipation, hemorrhoids, leg swelling, carpal tunnel syndrome, and difficulty sleeping due to this overall discomfort. About 10 percent of twin pregnancies become single pregnancies by the end of the first trimester as a result of spontaneous abortion (miscarriage) of one of the fetuses. Twin-twin transfusion also may occur.

Q. *What is twin-twin transfusion syndrome?*

A. One twin's placenta receives more blood flow than the other. This occurs in 20 percent of monochorionic diamniotic pregnancies, in less than 5 percent of overall twin pregnancies. The result: one twin is small and anemic and has low amniotic fluid (the "stuck" twin), and the other twin is much larger with normal or more amniotic fluid. This is usually seen in the second trimester. If untreated, the outcome is dismal, with a 90 percent mortality rate in the stuck twin and a 30 percent chance of a neurological handicap in the survivor. The treatment of choice is fetoscopic laser ablation of the intertwined blood vessels. Dual survivor rate is increased to at least 70 percent, with a decrease of neurological problems to 5 to 10 percent.

Q. *Will my prenatal care be different*
because I have a twin pregnancy?

A. You will be seeing your doctor much more frequently. You will also be seen by a perinatologist periodically throughout your pregnancy. Ultrasounds will be much more frequent. The ultrasounds will be performed to evaluate fetal growth and amniotic fluid levels. An ultrasound will also be performed to measure the length of your cervix to assess your risk of preterm labor. You will get routine NSTs in your third trimester to monitor the babies' health.

Q. *Are there any special instructions*
that I should follow if I am having twins?

A. Proper nutrition is even more important in a twin pregnancy. Weight gain should be increased to 40 pounds for the pregnancy. Usually, this is not a problem. Early weight gain is important for the growth of both babies. Moderate exercise before 28 weeks is recommended, with increased rest in the third trimester. Depending on your job, you may want to leave work on an early pregnancy disability leave. Sex has not been shown to increase the risk of preterm labor but may be too uncomfortable for you in your third trimester.

Q. *How will I deliver my twins?*

A. This will depend on the presentation of the twins at the time of labor and the philosophy of your doctor. At least 50 percent of the time, one or both babies are breech or in a transverse lie presentation, and a cesarean section will be advised. If one of the twins has FGR or low amniotic fluid, a C-section will be performed. Many times, the second baby cannot tolerate the labor contractions, in which case a C-section will be performed.

Q. *What is selective fetal reduction?*

A. Selective fetal reduction is the termination of one of the fetuses in a multiple-gestation pregnancy. This may be performed if the parents and physician decide that triplets, quadruplets, or more may be too risky a pregnancy for all the babies owing to the high likelihood of preterm labor and the decreased chance of survival of any of the newborns. This procedure may also be offered if there is a monochorionic twin pair with an increased risk of twin-twin transfusion or if one of the fetuses has a congenital defect that is incompatible with life and is endangering the well-being of the normal, healthy sibling(s). This procedure is usually not performed until the late first trimester. Once the pregnancy is reduced to twins, the prematurity rate decreases to the same as a nonreduced twin pregnancy, with an average birth age of 36 weeks.

STILLBIRTHS

Q. *How common are stillbirths?*

A. Stillbirths, or intrauterine fetal demise (IUFD), is luckily less than 5 per 1,000 births. The definition of IUFD is death of a fetus older than 20 weeks or weighing more than 500 grams (1pound, 2 ounces).

Q. *What are the risks factors for IUFD?*

A. The cause is unknown 50 percent of the time. Congenital and chromosomal abnormalities can by found 15 percent of the time. Lack of oxygen makes up the rest.

Predisposing factors include:

- Cocaine abuse
- Methamphetamine abuse
- Alcohol abuse
- Uncontrolled hypertension
- Uncontrolled diabetes
- Fetal growth restriction
- 41 weeks at delivery (triples the risk)
- 42 weeks at delivery (twelve times the risk)
- Advanced maternal age
- Multiple births

Q. *What happens if I have a stillborn?*

A. You may wait to go into spontaneous labor, which may not occur for weeks, or you may be induced or have an elective C-section. You will also be encouraged to request an autopsy, take photos of your baby, hold your baby, talk with your doctor, have a funeral service, and join a support group.

CHAPTER 9

Medical Complications of Pregnancy

Q. *How common is genital herpes in pregnancy?*

A. Almost 25 percent of pregnant women have had an outbreak of genital herpes or are positive for HSV-2 by blood test. Another 2 percent of pregnant women will contract genital herpes during pregnancy. If you have never had an outbreak of genital herpes but your partner has, your partner can get a blood test to see what type of HSV he has, and you should get tested to see if you have herpes, too.

Q. *What are the dangers of a primary genital herpes infection during pregnancy?*

A. If the infection occurs in the first trimester of pregnancy, there may be a slightly increased risk of miscarriage. Primary infection in the late second or in the third trimester has been associated with preterm delivery.

Q. *Can a primary infection of herpes during my pregnancy cause a congenital infection?*

A. A fetus with congenital malformations rarely if ever occurs because of a primary infection of herpes. Treatment is with the standard dose of herpes antiviral medications. These meds are category B and are safe to take during pregnancy. For symptomatic treatment, try sitz baths three to four times a day in soapy water with oatmeal soap and ask your doctor for a pain reliever, if needed.

Q. *What is the danger to my baby if I have a primary genital herpes infection when I go into labor and have a vaginal delivery?*

A. Approximately 50 percent of infants born vaginally to mothers with a primary vaginal herpes infection will have a herpes infection. Of these infected babies, about 60 percent will die within their first month of life. Of the survivors, 50 percent will have significant problems, such as seizures, an abnormally small head, mental retardation, small eyes, other eye problems, and meningitis. Remember, primary genital herpes infection in pregnancy is rare.

Q. *What is the danger to my baby if I have a recurrent genital herpes infection when I go into labor and have a vaginal delivery?*

A. It is estimated that only 4 percent of babies born vaginally to women who have a recurrent vaginal herpes infection will develop a herpes infection. The same risks, however, occur to these infected babies: 60 percent will die within the first month of life, and 50 percent of the survivors will have significant neurological disorders.

Q. *How can I make sure that I do not have or will not get genital herpes during my pregnancy?*

A. If you and your partner are unsure of your HSV status or if your partner is positive and you are unsure of your status, you may both be screened for HSV at your initial visit.

If you are both negative and monogamous, there are no worries. If you are positive for HSV, talk to your doctor about suppressive antiviral therapy at 36 weeks. If you are HSV negative and your partner is HSV positive, start using condoms during sex and refrain from sex in the third trimester. If your partner is HSV-1 positive or has cold sores, refrain from oral-genital contact, especially during the third trimester.

Q. *What will my doctor do if I have a history of genital herpes?*

A. Your doctor will prescribe an antiviral suppressive medication beginning at your 36th week. This will reduce your risk of both asymptomatic viral shedding and a recurrent outbreak at the time of delivery.

Q. *What should I do if I have an outbreak of herpes near term?*

A. Have a cesarean section. Even if you just have prodromal (just before) symptoms, such as burning, itching, or tingling in your legs, vulva, or vagina, have a cesarean section. This will prevent all possible chances of infection in your baby. If you have an active lesion when you go into labor or rupture your membranes, you will undergo a cesarean section. This should prevent a herpes infection in your infant more than 90 percent of the time.

With this plan of treatment, is not surprising that most women who deliver infants with herpes virus infections are unaware that they themselves are infected.

Q. *If I have an active herpes infection and a cesarean section, what will happen after delivery?*

A. You and your baby will be isolated during your hospital stay. You will be placed on antiviral suppressive therapy, which is safe to take while breast-feeding. Proper hygiene is recommended, including hand washing before you hold your baby. If you have an oral HSV outbreak, avoid kissing your baby until the lesion is cleared.

Q. *What are the signs and symptoms of a yeast infection?*

A. Yeast infections are caused by *Candida albicans*, a type of fungus that is normally found in your vagina. When the normal level of sugar increases or the acid-base balance is disturbed, the candida will thrive, overgrow, and cause the typical signs and symptoms of a yeast infection.

Signs and symptoms include a heavy vaginal discharge. The discharge is typically white and clumpy, giving it a cottage cheese appearance. On occasion, the discharge can be thick and iridescent green or yellow. The discharge may be odorless or have a faint yeast smell. Your vagina will feel itchy, irritated, or burning. The vagina may bleed if the irritation is intense. A yeast infection does not cause a miscarriage or preterm labor. The vulva may swell and feel warm and make sitting uncomfortable. Urinating may cause a stinging sensation in your vagina. Sex, if attempted, will be far from enjoyable.

Q. *Are yeast infections common during pregnancy?*

A. Up to 20 percent of pregnant women will develop a vaginal yeast infection, usually in the second or third trimester. Pregnancy is the most common predisposing factor for this infection.

Q. *Should I see my doctor if I have a yeast infection?*

A. Yes, other infections, such as STDs, cause similar symptoms which should be diagnosed and treated promptly.

Q. *What is the treatment for a*
yeast infection during pregnancy?

A. The same treatment applies whether you are pregnant or not. Preparations such as butoconozole nitrate (Femstat), butoconazole nitrate (Gynazole), clotrimazole (Gyne-Lotrimin, Mycelex-G) or terconazole (Terazol) all offer effective treatment. You may have to use the medication for a longer period of time (up to 2 weeks) to successfully control the overgrowth of candida; however, these medications are safe during pregnancy. Fluconazole (Diflucan), an oral treatment for yeast infections, has not yet been approved for treatment of yeast infections during pregnancy.

Q. *I took Diflucan in the first trimester before I*
realized that I was pregnant. What is the risk?

A. Although Diflucan has not been approved for use during pregnancy, its use during the first trimester has not caused an increase in birth defects or miscarriages.

Q. *What are the dangers of a yeast*
infection during pregnancy?

A. Babies born to women with yeast infections may develop thrush (an oral candida infection), a vaginal yeast infection, or diaper rash.

Q. *How can I prevent yeast infections?*

A. Always wipe front to back after urinating. Wear loose-fitting cotton underwear and change it frequently if it becomes damp. Change out of damp swim wear or gym clothes as soon as you are finished with your activity. Don't use perfumed or deodorant-containing sanitary pads, bubble baths, or feminine hygiene sprays.

Q. *What is a bacterial vaginosis (BV)?*

A. This is an infection caused by an overgrowth of many species of bacteria normally found in your vagina. One of the main bacterial species found in BV is *Gardnerella vaginalis*. BV is very common. Up to 25 percent of pregnant women may acquire a BV infection.

Q. *What causes BV in pregnancy?*

A. The overgrowth of bacteria is caused by an imbalance in certain types of bacteria. It is not an STD, but having sex can disturb the balance of bacteria in your vagina, making you more prone to BV. Most doctors screen for BV along with STDs during your first prenatal visit.

Q. *What are the signs and symptoms of BV?*

A. This infection produces a gray-white discharge that is foul smelling and, in a less acidic environment, may smell fishy. The fishy smell may become more apparent after intercourse owing to the presence of semen. However, many women have BV and have no signs or symptoms, which may lead to complications such as in increased risk of preterm labor if left untreated.

Q. *How is BV treated during pregnancy?*

A. BV may be safely treated throughout pregnancy with either oral or vaginal metronidazole or oral or vaginal clindamycin, whether you have symptoms or not, to prevent preterm labor.

Q. *Does BV cause any complications
during pregnancy?*

A. There is a concern that untreated BV may increase your risk for preterm labor (PTL) or premature rupture of membranes (PROM), especially in pregnant women with a past history of PTL.

Q. *What is a trichomonas infection?*

A. A trichomonad is a one-celled parasitic organism found in the vaginas of up to 15 percent of women without symptoms. The infection is sexually transmitted, so you could also be at risk for having another STD.

Q. *What are the signs and symptoms of
a trichomonas infection?*

A. When infection occurs, you will experience vaginal itching, swelling, or burning. The discharge will be a copious, fishy-smelling greenish or gray discharge.

Q. *What is the treatment for
trichomoniasis during pregnancy?*

A. Metronidazole is the treatment of choice for trichomoniasis during pregnancy. One recent large-scale study has shown that metronidazole does not cause an increase in birth defects when used at any time during your pregnancy. Metronidazole orally is the most effective treatment during pregnancy, but vaginal metronidazole can be used if the oral medicine is not tolerated. Your partner will be asymptomatic, but he needs to be treated if you want to have sex with him and not become reinfected.

Q. *Is a trichomonas infection*
dangerous during pregnancy?

A. There are suspicions that certain vaginal infections may increase the likelihood of preterm labor, and the efficacy of treatment of these infections in preventing preterm labor has not been established.

Q. *What is a venereal wart infection?*

A. Venereal warts, or *condylomata acuminata*, are caused by the human papillomavirus (HPV). They are acquired by sexual contact. These warts may grow on the vagina, vulva, perineum, anus, urethra, bladder, or cervix. Sometimes these warts grow and spread during pregnancy. This is a sexually transmitted disease (STD). There are many types of HPV. Some cause warts. Other subtypes cause abnormal Pap smears. The HPV infection is usually transmitted by an asymptomatic carrier.

This STD is really common—over 6 million new cases a year, mostly in teens and young adults in the United States. Easily over 25 million men and women have been infected with HPV. We now think that at least 75 percent of sexually active men and women will have a genital HPV infection sometime during their life.

Q. *Is there a cure for HPV infection?*

A. No cure. Only treatments. The good news is that your immune system can destroy the virus and eradicate it from your body—but this process can take one or more years.

Q. *How can venereal warts be prevented?*

A. Avoid skin-to-skin contact with a partner with HPV. Unfortunately, this may be hard to do because most men are asymptomatic carriers, and you cannot see the millions of submicroscopic viruses on his penis. Of course, most women will avoid sexual contact with a warty penis. Condoms cannot fully protect you from contracting HPV because there will be infected areas not covered by the condom. If you are in a monogamous relationship and you have HPV, so does your partner. If your warts disappear, don't worry about reinfection from your partner; this doesn't occur. There is an HPV vaccine that will be marketed soon that will immunize virgins from HPV-16, the most common sexually transmitted subtype.

Q. *How is a venereal wart
infection treated during pregnancy?*

A. For the usual small warts, treatment can be by cryosurgery (freezing), electrocautery (burning), acid destruction, or excision. These procedures are performed in your doctor's office.

Q. *What are the complications of a
venereal wart infection during pregnancy?*

A. Although extremely rare, these warts can grow to the size of golf balls during pregnancy. Also rare is growth of many new warts during your pregnancy. There have been reports of warts growing near or on the vocal cords of the infants if there is extensive disease and delivery is accomplished by the vaginal route. You may read something about this on the Internet. It is extremely rare. I have never seen it. You don't need a cesarean section to prevent a complication that is rare. Most commonly, these warts are small, few in number, easily removed, and do not cause complications during pregnancy or delivery.

Q. *What is a chlamydia infection?*

A. This is a sexually transmitted disease caused by bacteria called *Chlamydia trachomatis*. It may infect the cervix or cause salpingitis (inflammation of the tube). During pregnancy, only the cervix is infected, causing a yellowish discharge that may be scant and often goes unnoticed.

Q. *How can I prevent a chlamydia infection?*

A. Only have sex with a tested negative partner. Condom use will greatly reduce the risk of transmission.

Q. *Will I be tested for chlamydia during my pregnancy?*

A. Many doctors routinely test for chlamydia and gonorrhea at your first prenatal visit. Other doctors may screen only high-risk patients.

Q. *Can a chlamydia infection cause complications during pregnancy and problems for my baby after delivery?*

A. Yes, these pregnancies have a doubled risk for preterm birth. Up to 60 percent of babies will contract this infection after a vaginal delivery. A lesser percentage will become infected if a cesarean section was performed after membranes ruptured. Half of these infants may develop conjunctivitis if not treated with preventive erythromycin ointment, and 10 percent of babies may develop pneumonia, usually 6 weeks after delivery. There may also be an increased risk of ear and gastrointestinal infections in these babies.

Q. *What is the treatment for chlamydia infections during pregnancy?*

A. A single dose of azithromycin is the treatment of choice. Of course your partner(s) should be treated as well. A follow-up culture will be done a few months later.

Q. *What is giardiasis?*

A. Giardiasis is a disease caused by the parasite *Giardia lamblia*. The symptoms of this illness are fatigue, abdominal discomfort, and a bulky diarrhea with its own characteristic foul smell. Infection by giardia may come from drinking contaminated water from freshwater lakes, rivers, streams, ponds, swimming pools, hot tubs, or hot springs. Infection may also come from eating uncooked contaminated food or food prepared by a contaminated cook who did not wash his or her hands after a bowel movement. Giardia can also be found in surfaces that are contaminated, such as bathroom sinks and faucets, toilet seats, and public diaper-changing tables.

Q. *What is the effect of giardiasis on my pregnancy?*

A. There are no additional complications to your pregnancy. This parasite does not cross over the placenta to your fetus. You will just be more tired than usual and have more flatulence than usual as well as frequent greasy diarrheal stools that smell like burnt eggs.

Q. *What is the treatment of giardiasis during pregnancy?*

A. Giardiasis may be safely treated with metronidazole during pregnancy.

Q. *My child has pinworm, and I think I do, too. What should I do?*

A. Pinworm is caused by a parasite called *Enterobius vermicularis*. The usual symptoms are anal and vaginal itching. If symptoms are severe, treatment with pyrantel pamoate or pyrvinium pamoate is acceptable.

Q. *My Pap smear taken during my first prenatal visit came back abnormal. What does this mean?*

A. An abnormal Pap smear will occur in 5 to 10 percent of women, whether they are pregnant or not. An abnormal Pap smear means that some of the cells from your cervix were an irregular size or shape. Many times this may just be due to inflammation or infection. Infection of your cervix with the human papillomavirus (HPV) frequently causes abnormal Pap smears. The Pap smear has a 5 percent chance of a false positive or false negative result.

Q. *What will be done if I have an abnormal Pap smear during pregnancy?*

A. If your Pap smear is suspicious for an HPV infection, which may cause a precancerous lesion, your doctor will perform another office exam called *colposcopy*. This procedure is performed with a colposcope, an instrument that looks like binoculars with a multi-colored light source, through which your doctor will examine your cervix. Your cervix and vagina will be cleaned with a dilute solution of vinegar, and together with the different light sources and magnification, the normal and abnormal (if any) areas of your cervix will be clearly seen.

   If abnormal areas of cervix are identified, a biopsy of this tissue may be performed. There may be some amount of bleeding during this procedure; however, it is safe; there is no danger of a miscarriage or preterm labor. If the colposcopic exam reveals only normal tissue, no biopsy will be performed. The colposcopic exam will be repeated in 6 to 8 weeks, because during this time, the cervix will naturally evert, or turn inside out, a process that occurs gradually throughout your pregnancy. This will allow your doctor to see areas that were hidden before and that might contain a dysplastic lesion.

Q. *What will be done if I have a positive result from my biopsy?*

A. As long as the biopsy result shows mild dysplasia, colposcopic exams along with Pap smears will be performed throughout the remainder of your pregnancy. Treatment will be reserved for the postpartum period. If the biopsy is positive for cervical cancer, treatment may be performed during pregnancy after discussions with a cancer specialist.

Q. *What effects does pregnancy have on my asthma?*

A. Asthma is the most common chronic disease complicating a pregnancy. In fact, 5 to 8 percent of pregnant women have asthma. Pregnancy will generally improve your asthma symptoms during the first 29 weeks of your pregnancy. Then your asthma may worsen, remain the same, or improve even more. Everyone is different, and there is no way to predict how pregnancy may affect you. If the asthma does worsen, it is usually in the late second trimester and early third trimester. However, we do know that the effect on your asthma in one pregnancy will be the same in your subsequent pregnancies.

Q. *Will carrying a boy or girl affect my asthma?*

A. Yes. Being pregnant with a boy will make your breathing easier. It seems that the testosterone that your boy starts making at 8 weeks relaxes the bronchioles in your lungs.

Q. *What effect does my asthma have on my pregnancy?*

A. In the majority of pregnancies, if your asthma is well controlled by medication, there will be no complications. Poorly controlled asthma will lead to a lower oxygen supply to your baby, causing a small, undernourished baby (FGR). There may be a slight increase in preeclampsia.

Q. *What effect does asthma have on my baby?*

A. There is no increase in congenital defects in babies born to asthmatic mothers. Your baby does have a 6 percent chance of developing asthma during its first year of life and a 50 percent chance overall. If the father also has asthma, your baby's overall chance of developing asthma is about 75 percent.

Q. *Can I continue using the same asthma medications I was using before I became pregnant?*

A. Yes, you may use any of your asthma medications during pregnancy as prescribed by your doctor. They are safe for you and your baby.

Q. *Can I breast-feed if I am on asthma medication?*

A. Yes, breast-feeding is considered safe for women on asthma medication.

Q. *If I am a young breast cancer survivor, is it safe for me to get pregnant?*

A. Pregnancy is not a contraindication for breast cancer patients. In fact, the survival rates among breast cancer survivors is higher for those women who did become pregnant

Q. *How long should I wait after my treatment for breast cancer before I try to conceive?*

A. There is no right answer because no one really knows. The current recommendation is to wait between six and twenty-four months after treatment ends. Also, have your doctor perform a breast exam before you become pregnant or during your first or second prenatal visit.

Q. *What happens if my breast cancer is detected during my pregnancy?*

A. Most breast cancers detected during pregnancy are treated surgically with lumpectomy and axillary node dissection. The risks or benefits of additional therapy should be determined on a case-by-case basis. Radiation therapy in early pregnancy may cause fetal malformations, and later on in the pregnancy radiation exposure may cause fetal growth retardation and/or cancer in the newborn.

Chemotherapy in early pregnancy has a low (about 10 percent) risk of causing fetal malformations and in later pregnancy can cause growth retardation. Another route to take is to perform the surgery during pregnancy and then wait until after delivery to begin the other treatments. All these options depend on the trimester of pregnancy you are in, the type of breast cancer you have, and the stage of your breast cancer.

Q. *I have chronic hypertension and I am on medication. Should I stop taking it?*

A. No. If you have hypertension that required treatment before you conceived, you should continue to be treated during your pregnancy. Some of the hypertension medicines should be replaced with medicines that are preferred for use during pregnancy.

Q. *Which medicines should I be using for chronic hypertension during pregnancy?*

A. If you are planning your pregnancy, see your doctor to have baseline lab work and a possible change in medications. The two preferred medicines for treatment of chronic hypertension during pregnancy are methyldopa and labetalol. Both of these meds have been extensively studied during pregnancy and are safe for you and your baby.

Q. *Are there chronic hypertension medicines to avoid?*

A. ACE inhibitors are contraindicated during the second and third trimesters. Their use can cause kidney failure and fetal death. ACE inhibitors are safe during the first trimester for both mother and baby. So don't worry if you were taking this med in the beginning of your pregnancy before you realized that you were pregnant.

Q. *What effect does my chronic hypertension have on my pregnancy?*

A. Most women who have mild chronic hypertension before their pregnancies do well during their pregnancies, and their babies usually do well. Women with severe chronic hypertension before pregnancy have a high risk of having a baby with FGR, preeclampsia, and therefore (often) an induced preterm birth.

Q. *What is gestational diabetes?*

A. Gestational diabetes is diabetes that occurs during your pregnancy. Hormones from the placenta can decrease the activity of insulin and cause more glucose to appear in the blood. If your body cannot make enough insulin to drive the glucose into your cells for energy, there will be an increase in your blood glucose level.

Q. *How common is gestational diabetes?*

A. This condition occurs in about 5 percent of pregnancies.

Q. *When will I be screened for gestational diabetes?*

A. The recommended time interval for screening is between your 24th and 28th week of pregnancy. Your doctor may want to screen you at an earlier time if you have many high-risk factors.

Q. *How do I take the screening test for gestational diabetes?*

A. You will drink a very sugary drink and be advised to not eat or drink anything else for 1 hour. There is no need to fast beforehand. At 1 hour, a blood test will be performed to test your level of glucose. The drink can sometimes make you nauseous, so bring along some crackers to eat after your blood is drawn. If your glucose level is above the normal range, you still do not have gestational diabetes. This test is just a screening test. Your chances of having gestational diabetes if you "fail" this test are about 10 percent.

The next test will determine if your glucose control is really impaired. You will be asked to go to the lab in the morning before eating or drinking anything but water. A fasting blood glucose level will be drawn. You will then drink a larger amount of that sweet liquid (try another flavor this time) and will have blood taken 1, 2, and 3 hours later. Take a book; you have to stay in the lab. High glucose levels on this test give you the diagnosis of gestational diabetes.

Q. *Which women are more likely to get gestational diabetes?*

A. You may have an increased risk of acquiring gestational diabetes if you have one of the following conditions:

- Advanced maternal age
- Obesity
- Sedentary lifestyle
- Hypertension
- High cholesterol
- Polycystic ovarian syndrome
- Previous baby weighing at least 9 pounds
- Previous stillborn
- Family history of diabetes

About 10 percent of women with these risk factors will develop gestational diabetes. About 5 percent of women who don't have any of these risk factors may develop gestational diabetes. Therefore, all pregnant women are screened.

Q. *How is my gestational diabetes treated?*

A. You will be sent to a registered dietician who specializes in gestational diabetes. You will be counseled on your dietary habits and placed on a meal plan. You will be taught how to monitor your sugar levels with a glucometer and given the normal values to look for. An exercise regimen will be prescribed to help lower your glucose levels; follow it. You will review your progress with your dietician and physician periodically throughout the remainder of your pregnancy.

Q. *Will my doctor see me more frequently?*

A. You will be more closely monitored by your doctor. You may be referred to the perinatologist for a consult. You will have more ultrasounds to check the growth of your baby and the amount of amniotic fluid. NSTs will be done to monitor your baby's health. Your doctor will discuss the timing of your delivery and mode of delivery, which will depend on the size of your baby.

Q. *Do gestational diabetics ever develop insulin-requiring diabetes during pregnancy?*

A. About 10 percent of gestational diabetics will develop insulin-requiring diabetes. Therefore, it is important to monitor your sugar levels and follow the diet and exercise prescription.

Q. *What problems may occur in a pregnancy complicated by gestational diabetes?*

A. There is a higher incidence of bladder infections, preeclampsia, polyhydramnios (too much amniotic fluid), and macrosomia. In macrosomia, the baby weighs more than 9 pounds. A macrosomic infant has an increased chance of causing a difficult labor complicated by arrest of cervical dilation and long hours of pushing without successful descent of the baby, requiring cesarean section. Sometimes the baby's large shoulders are difficult to deliver, which can cause trauma to both you and your newborn. By following the diet and exercise program your doctor prescribes, you will be able to deliver a healthy infant.

Q. *What do I do postpartum?*

A. After the placenta is delivered, you can have a chocolate cake! Your glucose metabolism is back to normal. Following a healthy diet and continuing to exercise, since you're in the habit of doing so, is a wise move.

Q. *What is mitral valve prolapse (MVP)?*

A. MVP is a minor abnormality of the mitral valve in your heart. The valve is usually very large and has excessive tissue. The diagnosis is confirmed by an ultrasound of your heart called an *echocardiogram.*

Q. *What are the symptoms of MVP?*

A. Usually you will have no symptoms, but if you do, the most common symptoms are palpitations and chest pain. Other complaints may include shortness of breath, fatigue, and anxiety—also common complaints of pregnancy.

Q. *How will MVP affect my pregnancy?*

A. Most women do fine during their pregnancy, without any complications.

Q. *Will my doctor take any special precautions during my labor?*

A. It is recommended that doctors administer prophylactic antibiotics to women in labor if the mitral valve prolapse is complicated by mitral insufficiency (regurgitation) as well.

Q. *What can I take if I have a common cold?*

A. If your symptoms are very mild, try drinking large amounts of fluid. This will thin out the mucus in your nose or lungs and relieve the "stuffy" feeling. A vaporizer or humidifier may also help. When you sleep at night, prop yourself up on a few pillows to drain the mucus from your nose and enable you to breathe more easily. Sore throats may be soothed by gargling with warm salt water and using a throat spray or lozenges. Before you plan on taking any medication during pregnancy, contact your doctor.

Q. *What causes the common cold?*

A. Viruses. Rhinovirus is the cause of about 35 percent of colds during the spring, summer, and early fall. Coronoviruses cause the winter and early spring colds.

Q. *Will a cold harm my baby?*

A. No. There is no evidence that the common cold causes any birth defects or harms your baby.

Q. *What should I do if I have a fever?*

A. You should notify your doctor if you have a temperature above 100.4°F. If you have a high fever and flu symptoms, take acetaminophen (Tylenol, Datril, or Panadol) to lower your temperature, drink plenty of fluids to replenish what you have lost in perspiration, and stay in bed and rest.

Q. *What are the symptoms of the flu?*

A. The flu is a viral respiratory illness caused by the influenza viruses. Symptoms include high fevers, headache, sore throat, dry cough, runny/stuffy nose, fatigue, and muscle aches.

Q. *How doe the flu spread?*

A. The flu spreads from infected droplets released from coughing or sneezing. The infected droplets can even be passed by touching something that was sprayed with droplets and then touching your nose or mouth. A person with the flu may infect others beginning 1 day before they develop symptoms, before they are sick, and up to 5 days after becoming sick.

Q. *What are the dangers of an influenza
viral infection during pregnancy?*

A. Pregnant women are at increased risk for complications of the flu. Your immune system is weaker and cannot effectively fight off the infection. Your heart is working harder already, and your lung size is decreased from your pregnancy. These changes contribute to an almost double the risk of hospitalization in the first half of your pregnancy and a fourfold risk of being hospitalized in the second half of your pregnancy. The complications can be dehydration, pneumonia, and heart failure.

Q. *Should I get the flu vaccine?*

A. You should receive the flu vaccine if you are pregnant between October to mid-May to prevent yourself from getting the flu. The flu shot is composed of three types of inactivated (dead) viruses.

Q. *Can I get the flu vaccine in
     my first trimester?*

A. Yes. The flu shot does not cause an infection in your baby. The flu shot does not cause birth defects. The flu shot will not cause any pregnancy complications if administered in any trimester.

Q. *If my due date is October 8,
     should I still get the flu vaccine?*

A. Yes. Being immunized to the flu virus will immunize you and your newborn. Your baby will be born with your antibodies to the flu. This is important for your baby because newborns up to age six months don't make their own antibodies in response to the vaccine and will otherwise be unprotected.

Q. *What are the side effects
     of the flu vaccine?*

A. The most common side effect is soreness at the site of the shot. It is rare for adults to have a flu-like reaction after the shot.

Q. *What is a cytomegalovirus (CMV) infection?*

A. CMV is a viral infection. At least 95 percent of the time the infection is asymptomatic. The remaining 5 percent of infected individuals have a mononucleosis-like illness (fever, fatigue, sore throat, muscle pain, and lymph node enlargement) that may last from 1 week to 2 months. The virus can be passed through infected saliva, urine, feces, and breast milk. Primary CMV infection occurs in 0.7 to 4 percent of pregnant women.

Q. *Who is at high risk for contracting a CMV infection?*

A. Pregnant women who work at day-care centers, elementary school teachers, special education teachers, or moms with young children are at high risk.

Q. *How do I know if I have developed a CMV infection during pregnancy?*

A. Because the viral infection rarely causes symptoms, it is hard to diagnose. But if there is a known outbreak where you work or live, and if you do have symptoms of an infection, and if your fundal height growth has lagged, an ultrasound may reveal oligohydramnios, FGR, and swelling of your baby's tissues. An amniocentesis and culture will lead to the diagnosis.

Q. *What are the effects of a congenital CMV infection?*

A. Severe disease will occur in 80 to 90 percent of infected infants. These babies may have hearing loss, visual problems, mental or motor retardation, or behavior problems. The disease is fatal in a minority of those infants infected. About 10 percent of babies will be born without symptoms but will subsequently develop some degree of hearing loss, mental impairment, and coordination problems.

Q. *If I had a CMV infection before my pregnancy but was reinfected during my pregnancy, can I pass the infection to my fetus?*

A. Yes, but only 1 percent of the time. The infection in your baby is uniformly mild with no symptoms during the pregnancy or at birth, with mild hearing loss developing later as an infant.

Q. *If my blood tests showed that I was immune to German measles (rubella), should I worry if I am exposed to a child with this disease?*

A. No. If you are immune, you have already had rubella and you have antibodies in your blood to prevent another infection. At least 85 percent of women are immune by age twenty, and almost 100 percent by age thirty-five. Many states require a blood test for rubella before obtaining a marriage certificate, and if you are not immune, your doctor will advise you to get the vaccine.

Q. *If I was not immune to rubella and was exposed to the disease, what will happen to my baby?*

A. Congenital rubella infection is most devastating when the pregnant woman contracts the disease in the first trimester; up to

50 percent of the infants may become infected. Later on in pregnancy, only about 15 percent of infants will show evidence of infection. These babies may have cataracts, deafness, or mental retardation. Luckily, since mass vaccination of children began over twenty years ago, congenital rubella has become very rare.

Q. *I received a rubella vaccine before I realized that I was pregnant. How will my baby be affected?*

A. The rubella vaccine is a live virus and is not recommended during pregnancy. Furthermore, it is advised to wait three months before becoming pregnant. Of the fetuses inadvertently exposed to the rubella vaccine, only 2 percent had the virus at birth. Not one of the babies, however, showed signs of congenital anomalies. Termination of pregnancy only because of a rubella vaccination is not recommended.

Q. *If I had chicken pox as a child, should I worry if I come into contact with an individual who has chicken pox?*

A. No. If you had chicken pox, you cannot contract this viral disease again.

Q. *I don't know if I had chicken pox or the varicella-zoster virus (VZV) vaccine. What should I do?*

A. At least 70 to 90 percent of women who can't recall having chicken pox as a child will have antibodies showing previous infection. The vaccine has been out since 1995, so many of you moms will have been vaccinated. If you never had chicken pox, you can get the vaccine. You must wait one month after the second shot before you conceive.

Q. *If I have never had chicken pox and am exposed, what effects will it have on me and my fetus?*

A. The occurrence of congenital malformations due to chicken pox is very rare. The risk of congenital birth defects if exposed in the first trimester is 1 percent, and 2 percent in the second trimester. The abnormalities caused by this infection can be a small head, severe learning disabilities, blindness, growth problems, limb deformities, and scars. Chicken pox infection at term may be complicated by a severe pneumonia in the mom.

Q. *Is there treatment for chicken pox during pregnancy?*

A. If you have not had chicken pox, you should be immunized with varicella-zoster immune globulin (VZIG) within 4 days of exposure to the infected person. The benefit of VZIG is a reduction in the severity of your illness. Congenital infection is not prevented with VZIG. The use of oral acyclovir will also reduce your symptoms but will not prevent birth defects.

Q. *What is shingles?*

A. Shingles, also called *herpes zoster*, is caused by the chicken pox virus that had been dormant in your nerve root ever since your infection. You will get painful blisters in a strip of skin on only one side of your body.

Q. *Is shingles contagious?*

A. Yes, but only if you have never had chicken pox. It is possible to get shingles if you had the VZV vaccine, but it is really very unlikely. The infection is transmitted by contact with the lesion and only rarely by saliva.

Q. *What is fifth disease?*

A. Fifth disease is a viral infection characterized by a "slapped cheek" red rash on the face and a red body rash with maybe a slight fever in a child. An adult will have the rash, fever, and joint pain. Twenty percent of infections are asymptomatic. This is a childhood disease. At least 50 percent of adults have had the disease as a child.

Q. *What causes fifth disease?*

A. Fifth disease is caused by a virus called parvovirus B19. The virus is transmitted by respiratory secretions and hand-to-mouth contact. This infection can be spread for about 10 days after being exposed, but once the rash appears, the person is no longer infectious.

Q. *Who is at high risk of being exposed to fifth disease?*

A. The greatest risk of infection with parvovirus B19 is from your children; you'll have a 50 percent chance. Teachers have a 20 to 50 percent chance of infection.

Q. *I am pregnant and exposed to fifth disease.*
   What should I do?

A. A blood test can be performed to see if you have ever had a past infection or if you have not had a past infection and did or did not become infected. If you have evidence of a past infection, there is nothing to do. If you did not become infected, you will want to avoid further chances of exposure. If you have been exposed, discuss the options with your doctor.

Q. *I have been infected with parvovirus B19.*
   What will happen to my baby?

A. The transmission of the virus to your baby is between 20 and 33 percent, so there will be no problems in at least two-thirds of the babies. Infected babies do not have birth defects. The infection can cause swelling in the tissues in your baby, called *hydrops fetalis*, a miscarriage, or stillbirths. The risk is greatest if the infection occurs before your 20th week. The complications, if they do occur, will be evident by 8 weeks. If there is no hydrops by then, your baby will be fine with no long-term abnormalities.

Q. *How will my pregnancy be monitored?*

A. Weekly ultrasounds will be performed to monitor the health of your baby.

Q. *What is hand, foot, and mouth*
   disease (HFMD)?

A. HFMD is caused by a virus called *Coxsackie A16* or some other enteroviruses. It is a common childhood illness. The illness begins with a mild fever and sore throat. A day or two later, painful blisters start to appear in your mouth. Then a skin rash located on your palms and soles appear that is raised and red. The rash does not itch.

Q. *What happens if I am exposed to HFMD during my pregnancy?*

A. You may have a very mild illness if at all. There will be no harmful effects to your baby during your pregnancy. If infected just before you deliver, your baby may have a mild illness.

Q. *Are urinary tract infections (UTIs) common in pregnancy?*

A. Infection of the bladder and/or kidney(s) is the most common infection during pregnancy. A UTI may occur in up to 3 percent of pregnancies in middle- or upper-class women and in up to 10 percent of those in lower economic classes. The infection may or may not produce symptoms.

Q. *How will I know if I have a bladder infection (cystitis)?*

A. You may experience one or all of these symptoms: an increased frequency of urination (perhaps every 10 minutes), an increased urge to urinate, pain or cramps in your abdomen just above your pubic bone, difficulty beginning to urinate, a burning with urination. Your urine may look cloudy or there may be blood or mucus present. Your urine may have a different strong smell or a foul smell. If you have any one of these symptoms, tell your doctor, who will then examine your urine more closely. Remember, you may have these symptoms as a normal result of being pregnant.

Q. *How is cystitis treated?*

A. There are several different antibiotics that may be safely used during pregnancy. In addition, be sure to drink at least eight glasses of fluid a day to help flush the bacteria out of your bladder.

Q. *What is asymptomatic bacteriuria?*

A. This is a bladder infection with a small concentration of bacteria, so small that you do not have any signs or symptoms of a bladder infection.

Q. *What is the significance of asymptomatic bacteriuria?*

A. If left untreated, you have up to a 25 percent chance of getting a kidney infection. That is one reason why we check your urine at each prenatal visit.

Q. *Will a bladder infection harm my pregnancy?*

A. The only potential danger is that you may develop a kidney infection if you are not treated.

Q. *How will I know if I have a kidney infection (pyelonephritis)?*

A. Fortunately, kidney infections are less common than bladder infections, but they are the most common of the serious infections that occur during pregnancy. When they do occur, they are more common on the right side. The most common symptoms are flank pain, fever of 101°F or higher, chills, nausea and vomiting, and/or symptoms of cystitis.

Q. *How is pyelonephritis treated?*

A. Treatment is best initiated by hospitalization. You will receive an IV for two reasons: First, you may be very dehydrated from high fever and excessive perspiration and vomiting. Second, antibiotic treatment through an IV is the treatment of choice. With this treatment, 90 percent of patients will feel better within 1 to 2 days, and treatment can then be continued at home with oral antibiotics.

Q. *Is a kidney infection harmful to my pregnancy?*

A. If left untreated, pyelonephritis may cause premature labor.

Q. *Can surgery be safely performed during pregnancy?*

A. Yes. Although the need for surgery does not arise too often, if surgery must be performed, you and your fetus will in most instances not be adversely affected.

Q. *What are the most common reasons for surgery during pregnancy?*

A. The most common operations are for emergency situations: appendicitis, ovarian cysts, gallbladder disease, broken bones, or dental emergencies.

Q. *How common is appendicitis
    during pregnancy?*

A. Appendicitis occurs in about 1 in 2,000 pregnancies.

Q. *How common are ovarian cysts
    during pregnancy?*

A. Up to 4 percent of pregnant women will be diagnosed with an
ovarian cyst.

Q. *What are the symptoms of an ovarian cyst?*

A. Most of the time you will be unaware that you have an ovarian cyst. Your doctor may discover a cyst during the pelvic exam or
ultrasound on your first prenatal visit. Even very large cysts, like
the size of a softball, will go unnoticed. Symptoms will occur if the
cyst twists on its blood supply (torsion), which will cause sudden
excruciating pain. Fortunately, this happens very rarely.

Q. *What is the most common
    ovarian cyst in pregnancy?*

A. The majority of ovarian cysts are corpus luteum cysts of pregnancy, which almost always resolve spontaneously by the end of
the first trimester.

Q. *I have an ovarian cyst that is the size of
    a tennis ball. What will my doctor do?*

A. If the cyst is fluid filled and you have no symptoms, nothing
but serial ultrasounds will be done during your pregnancy.

Endometriomas may be observed throughout your pregnancy without the need for surgery. If the cyst is solid, there is still little to worry about. Most cysts can be correctly identified as benign by ultrasound or MRI. If you are going to have a C-section for some other indication, the cyst can be safely removed at that time. If the cyst is still present on your postpartum exam, surgery can be scheduled.

Q. *What is the treatment for an ovarian cyst that is suspicious for cancer?*

A. First of all, this is a rare occurrence in pregnancy. If there is a question of a possible ovarian cancer, surgery should be performed with a gynecological cancer specialist. The surgery can safely be performed either by laparoscopy or laparotomy.

Q. *Should I have elective surgery during pregnancy?*

A. Although such surgery is usually safe during pregnancy, I do not advise elective surgery, such as cosmetic surgery, being performed during this time.

Q. *What is the definition of normal weight?*

A. The BMI, or body mass index, is used to define weight. There are four categories of BMI:

- Underweight, < 18.5
- Normal weight, 18.5–24.9
- Overweight, 25–29.9
- Obesity, >30

If you want to calculate your BMI, go online to: cdc.gov/nccdphp/dnpa/bmi.

Q. *I calculated my BMI and I am obese,*
but I still want to get pregnant now.
What are my risks due to my weight?

A. Obese women have a greater risk of prepregnancy diabetes and hypertension, miscarriage, gestational diabetes, preeclampsia, fetal macrosomia (large babies), shoulder dystocia, and babies with neural tube defects. There is a higher rate of C-sections in obese women. Placement of an epidural or spinal for anesthesia may be more challenging, as is intubation if general anesthesia is performed. Cesarean sections on obese moms can be complicated by a greater blood loss, a longer surgery time, postoperative blood clots in the legs, and a higher rate of infections of the uterus and skin incision.

Q. *Are obese women at increased risk of*
having a baby with a birth defect?

A. Yes. The risk of neural tube defects such as spina bifida or anencephaly is twice as common in babies born to obese women.

Q. *I had bariatric surgery.*
When is it safe to get pregnant?

A. You should wait at least twelve to eighteen months. This is the time period when your body will be in the rapid weight loss phase.

Q. *Do I have increased nutritional requirements after bariatric surgery?*

A. You will need additional supplements of iron, vitamin B_{12}, folic acid, and calcium.

Q. *Are there increased risks to my pregnancy after bariatric surgery?*

A. No. Women who have had bariatric surgery and are not obese do as well as other women of the same weight. If you have had gastric banding, an adjustment may be needed during your pregnancy.

CHAPTER 10

Labor and Delivery

Q. *Is it common to be nervous about going into labor?*

A. Absolutely. Whether it is your first or fourth, this is a major stressful event. Let's discount pain for now because you can have an epidural whenever you want. You are going to give birth to a new life that you helped create and will care for. This is a major responsibility—the most important that you have.

Q. *What is labor?*

A. Labor is the occurrence of regular uterine contractions that bring about a change in the cervix—effacement and dilation—allowing your baby to be delivered vaginally.

Q. *What is effacement?*

A. Effacement, which actually may begin before labor, is the thinning of your cervix. The cervix, when not effaced, is from 1 to 2 inches thick. When completely effaced, it is as thin as paper. Effacement is described as a percentage; complete effacement is 100 percent. The percentages between 0 and 100 are subjective but still reproducible among experienced examiners.

Q. *What is dilation?*

A. Dilation is the progressive widening of your cervical opening. It is measured in centimeters. A completely dilated cervix is 10 centimeters, wide enough to allow passage of your baby into the birth canal, your vagina. Dilation may begin before labor, too. Many women may begin labor already dilated 1 to 5 centimeters. Measurement of your cervical dilation is subjective.

Q. *What is station?*

A. This refers to the level of the baby's head in relation to the ischial spines, a bony protuberance located in the pelvis and easily felt by your doctor or nurse during the pelvic exam. The head felt at the level of the spines is at 0 station. If the head is above this level ("floating"), then a minus value is given, from -1 to -3. A positive value is assigned when the head is below the spines, from $+1$ to $+3$, then "crowning." This is also a reproducible subjective measurement.

Q. *What is engagement?*

A. Engagement, or "lightening," refers to the drop of your baby's head into your pelvis. With your first pregnancy, this may occur a few weeks before the onset of labor. When it occurs suddenly, you may notice it. You will be aware of an increased pressure in your pelvis and vagina, increased frequency to urinate, easier breathing with less pressure on your rib cage, and less heartburn. With subsequent pregnancies, engagement usually occurs with the start of labor.

Q. *What is "show" or "bloody show"
or the "mucous plug"?*

A. This is a mucous or blood-tinged mucous discharge from the vagina. The mucous plug, which filled the cervical canal, has dislodged. This may occur within hours of labor or two weeks before labor begins or only after labor has begun.

Q. *What should I do if I lose my mucous plug?*

A. Not a thing. Don't save it for your doctor. Don't call your doctor. It is not an emergency. It means that you will probably go into labor within two weeks. Are you ready?

Q. *What is a ripe cervix?*

A. This is a condition in which the cervix is soft, at least 50 percent effaced, and 2 or more centimeters dilated, and the head is engaged, closely applied to the cervix, and at least a -2 station.

Q. *What is crowning?*

A. The vagina and perineum are distended, and about 1 inch of the baby's head is visible in between contractions.

Q. *What is Pitocin?*

A. Pitocin, or "pit," is a synthetic form of oxytocin, a hormone produced by the pituitary gland in your brain. Pitocin is given intravenously, if needed, to stimulate uterine contractions. It causes the muscles in the uterus to contract more frequently and with a greater intensity. The effects of Pitocin begin working within minutes and last only a few minutes when given through an IV, so the strength and frequency of the contractions can be accurately controlled.

Q. *What are the possible complications of using Pitocin?*

A. Pitocin is a very potent medication. The infusion of Pitocin is started at a very low concentration by a metered infusion pump. Raising the infusion rate after timed intervals and only if necessary will rarely cause an untoward side effect. Rarely, hyperstimulation of the uterus may occur. This may cause a prolonged contraction or uterine contractions that occur immediately one after the other. The result is a decreased blood flow to the fetus and decreased oxygen to the fetus. Stopping the infusion of the Pitocin reverses these complications within minutes. Terbutaline may also be given to reverse the effects.

Q. *What is a birthing bed?*

A. The birthing bed is one of the truly great advances for the woman in labor. This bed at first glance appears to be your normal hospital bed with all the modern conveniences: electronic controls to raise the head or foot of the bed and wheels. The added modification is the charm. The mattress at the foot of the bed may be taken off and stirrups may be placed at this end to convert the laboring bed to a delivery bed. This is all done in the labor, delivery, and postpartum suite.

Q. *What is a prep?*

A. The nurse shaves the pubic hair located between the bottom of your vagina and the top of your anus (the perineum), the area where an episiotomy might be performed and repaired. I haven't seen a nurse do a prep in fifteen years. You can go for a wax or trim at your local spa anytime during your pregnancy if you so desire.

Q. *Why is an enema ordered?*

A. The enema is used to evacuate your rectum and lower intestines. This may come as a relief to some women who have been constipated, sensed a pressure in their pelvis, and do not want to have a bowel movement when they are pushing. Many women have had loose stools or diarrhea before entering the hospital and may not need an enema. Discuss the use of enemas with your doctor. Once again, it's been about fifteen years since doctors routinely ordered enemas.

Q. *What are Braxton Hicks contractions?*

A. False labor, or Braxton Hicks contractions, are irregular contractions of your uterus. These contractions may occur at any time during your pregnancy, but they become more common near term. However, you may never experience them. These uterine contractions can last from 5 seconds to 2 minutes, but usually last 30 to 45 seconds. The discomfort from these contractions can be felt in your back, front, down low in your pelvis, just on one side, or even in one isolated spot near the top of your uterus. Most commonly the pain is experienced in the front of your uterus.

Q. *How can I tell the difference between Braxton Hicks contractions and labor?*

A. Braxton Hicks contractions are usually irregular in the duration of the contraction or irregular in the interval between contractions. Real labor contractions can start out at irregular intervals but become regular over time. The duration of the contraction is regular, lasting 45 to70 seconds.

Braxton Hicks contractions usually stop or become less intense with a change in your position. For example, if you notice them while sitting or lying down, get up and walk around and the contractions will fade. Real labor contractions will remain at regular intervals despite a change in activity. Braxton Hicks contractions may be perceived as strong but will weaken over a few hours. Real labor contractions may initially be perceived as weak but will gain strength over time. Braxton Hicks contractions most commonly occur in the evening. Real labor contractions can start anytime day or night.

Q. *Thanks for the explanation, but what if I'm still not sure if I'm in early labor?*

A. Occasionally, first-time pregnant women and even veterans cannot tell the difference between false and real labor. See your doctor if you are unsure. If it is after office hours, go to labor and delivery (L&D) to be monitored for uterine contractions and have your cervix checked. Sometimes it takes a few hours to determine if you are in labor. If you come in with preterm labor, a fetal fibronectin test will be done. Remember, the definition of labor is the progressive dilation of your cervix. Don't feel embarrassed if this happens more than once; some women must be checked for false labor two or more times near term.

Remember, false labor pains are mild, irregular, last 30 to 45 seconds, are not accompanied by an increased flow of mucus from your vagina, and usually disappear with a change in your position.

Q. *How do I know that I am in labor?*

A. The signs of labor are regular contractions lasting 45 to 90 seconds, often but not always with the appearance of a mucous discharge (mucous plug) that can be mixed with blood (bloody show) and/or leaking of amniotic fluid. The contractions often begin at intervals of 15 to 20 minutes, are mild, and may last only 30 seconds. The contractions may occur at this time interval for several hours, or the interval may shorten to 5 minutes within 1 hour. The former usually occurs with your first pregnancy, the latter with a subsequent pregnancy. It is possible that the contractions may begin at 5 minutes apart, especially if you had a quick labor course with a previous pregnancy.

Q. *Does the baby move during labor?*

A. Labor does not quiet down the actions of your fetus. He or she will still kick and roll during your labor. If you notice a decrease in your baby's activity during early labor at home, go to labor and delivery to be monitored.

Q. *Is it normal to have diarrhea at the beginning of labor?*

A. Yes. Some of the hormonal changes that occur at the onset of labor may provoke diarrhea in some women.

Q. *When should I go to the hospital?*

A. Discuss this with your doctor. In general, I advise my patients to go to labor and delivery when their contractions are 5 minutes apart, lasting 1 minute, and have been timed for 1 hour. I also advise my patients to go to L&D if their contractions are 6 or 7 minutes apart but are becoming so painful that they are thinking that pain relief from an epidural is a good idea. Time the contractions from the beginning of one contraction to the beginning of the next. You should also go to L&D if your membranes have ruptured (if your water has broken) or if you think that your membranes have ruptured even if you are not in labor. If you had a previous rapid labor (less than 4 hours), go to L&D when your contractions are 8 to 10 minutes apart for 1 hour; they may be 3 minutes apart the next hour, and you could deliver at home or en route, especially if you live far from the hospital. Do not have anything to eat once labor begins. Remember, drive safely to the hospital; don't speed or drive through red lights.

Q. *What happens when I get to the hospital?*

A. Go to the admitting desk. Be sure to preregister at the hospital; making financial arrangements and filling out forms while you are in labor, especially in the middle of the night, can be frustrating. You will then be taken by wheelchair to the labor and delivery area.

Q. *What are the initial procedures*
in labor and delivery?

A. You are greeted by a nurse who will show you to your room. You will be asked to change into a hospital gown and supply a sample of urine. Your urine will be tested for the presence of sugar, protein, and ketones. You will be asked to get into your labor bed. The external monitors will be placed for listening to your baby's heart and monitoring your contractions. The nurse will perform a vaginal exam, record your blood pressure, temperature, and pulse, and observe for signs of labor. The nurse will then call your doctor to relay the information gathered and to receive instructions and orders.

Q. *What may the doctor order?*

A. Standard orders include external fetal monitoring, pain medication as needed, instructions that the patient may or may not get out of bed, blood tests, IV only when indicated, oral fluids, or special medications (for preexisting conditions).

Q. *What does the labor room look like?*

A. Labor rooms in most private hospitals have one labor bed in each room. The rooms are nicely decorated with patterned wallpaper, pictures, nightstands, a telephone, and a television set. It is decorated to have a "homey," comfortable atmosphere. Many rooms will have a day bed for your partner or labor coach. There is an intercom, so you may call your nurse. There will be a fetal monitor in the room and a hookup for oxygen, if needed. You will have a private bathroom with a shower.

Q. *When does the doctor come to the hospital?*

A. This really depends on the time of day (or night) you arrive at the hospital, the stage of labor you are in, and whether it is your first labor or your second or more. If you are admitted in the middle of the night and you are in the early stages of labor, your doctor will see you in the morning. If you are admitted from the office, the doctor will see you after office hours. If this is your first pregnancy, the doctor will come to the hospital after you have started pushing; if you've had a previous birth, the doctor will arrive when you are in the active phase if you don't have an epidural, with the onset of pushing if you do have an epidural. Of course, if there are any complications, your doctor will be notified and will be at L&D right away.

Q. *What are the stages of labor?*

A. There are three stages of labor. In the first stage, divided into a latent phase and an active phase, the cervix dilates to 10 centimeters. In the second stage, the baby descends through the birth canal and is delivered. In the third stage, the placenta is expelled.

Q. *What happens during the latent phase?*

A. This is the beginning of labor. Your contractions change from being irregular and 15 to 20 minutes apart to 5 to 6 minutes apart. During this phase, the cervix begins to dilate and efface. If this is your first pregnancy, your cervix at the start of labor may be undilated and uneffaced. If this is a subsequent pregnancy, you may begin this phase with cervix dilated from 1 to 5 centimeters and almost completely effaced. The average length of the latent phase is 6 to 7 hours for a primiparous (first-time) patient and 4 to 5 hours for a multiparous patient. The baby will descend from a −2 to a 0 station. Your contractions will last longer and will feel more uncomfortable near the end of this phase. Usually your membranes are intact (your water has not broken). Most women can carry on conversations, read, watch television, or walk. Many women get to the hospital near the end of this phase.

Q. *How long can the latent phase last?*

A. A prolonged latent phase may last more than 20 hours in the primiparous and 14 hours in the multiparous patient.

Q. *What happens if I have a*
prolonged latent phase?

A. The doctor may give you a sedative or a pain reliever to permit you to sleep; 85 percent of women will awake in the active phase, 10 percent will cease contracting (false labor), and 5 percent may require Pitocin.

Q. *What happens during the active phase?*

A. Your cervix is 4 to 5 centimeters dilated and 100 percent effaced. Contractions are now stronger, lasting 45 to 90 seconds and 2 to 3 minutes apart. You are in the transition stage, and the intensity of the contractions has now become extremely uncomfortable. You may not feel like talking now and may become irritable; your sense of humor may be all but lost. The contractions may be quite painful now. The contraction pain may be felt in the front or in the back. The pain may radiate (travel) down to your rectum or thighs. The pain may be strong but bearable or sharp, cramping, aching, throbbing, and shooting with pressure. This is the time to employ your coping mechanisms that you have practiced, or you may ask for narcotic medication or an epidural. You probably will want to remain in bed and find a comfortable position, although most women will change position often during this stage. The baby descends to a +2 station near the end of the first stage. Some women may have the bearing-down sensation or feel like moving their bowels when only 6 to 9 centimeters. If this is your first pregnancy, concentrate on your breathing or relaxation techniques, and if you feel the need, ask for pain medication to dull this sensation. Pushing against a partially dilated cervix may lengthen this phase by causing swelling of the cervix and partial closing of the opening. Many multiparas (women who have delivered more than one child) may push the cervix from 8 centimeters to complete (10 centimeters) without difficulty and enter the second stage.

Q. *How long does the active phase last?*

A. The active phase usually lasts from 2 to 4 hours. It may be less than 1 hour in a multipara.

Q. *Are there certain positions I can be in to speed up my labor?*

A. No. There is no position that is better than another to speed up labor. Many women may want to walk around in early labor but will quickly return to bed at the onset of active labor. In the early part of the active phase, most women will prefer to lie on their side or recline in the sitting position in bed. Most women will naturally curl up in the fetal position during the end of the active stage when the contractions are the most intense. This answer applies to women who choose not to have an epidural.

Q. *Will a hot shower or lying in a hot tub speed up my labor?*

A. No. It will not speed up labor, prevent prolonged labor, or prevent or cause an indication for a cesarean section.

Q. *What happens if my active phase is prolonged?*

A. You will be stuck at certain dilation (for example, 6 centimeters) for more than 2 hours. If your membranes are still intact, artificial rupture of your membranes may strengthen the intensity of your contractions. An internal uterine pressure catheter (IUPC) will then be placed to monitor the strength and duration of your contractions. If the contractions are still weak or the interval is still greater than 3 minutes apart and your cervical exam is the same, you will need Pitocin. At this point, an IV will be started and Pitocin will be administered. Cervical dilation will resume within 2 hours in 85 percent of patients if labor was normal before the arrest of dilation. If progress does not ensue, you will have a cesarean section.

Q. *Can an epidural slow the progress of labor?*

A. Sometimes an epidural can increase the length of labor by less than 2 hours if given in early labor. If the interval of your contractions has lengthened to less than three per 10 minutes or their intensity has decreased, your doctor may give you Pitocin.

Q. *Can intense pain cause an arrest of dilation?*

A. Yes. Sometimes the pain can be so intense that a woman will involuntarily push against the cervix multiple times, causing the tissues of the cervix to swell and not dilate. Pain relief, especially an epidural in this case, will allow this individual to relax. Within a short time, the cervical swelling will disappear and cervical dilation can resume.

Q. *What happens during the second stage of labor?*

A. Your baby's head is now in the birth canal (your vagina) at a +2 station. It is time to push your baby out.

Q. *What is "laboring down"?*

A. Once you are completely dilated (10 centimeters), you may or may not have the urge to push if you have had an epidural. If you do not have the urge to push and a trial of pushing does not significantly move your baby's head down the birth canal, you will be allowed to labor down while the anesthesiologist adjusts the anesthetic. There may be an hour of waiting until you can feel the pressure of your baby's head and an urge to push. During this time, the baby's head may advance down your birth canal. If you are a rookie, the head may not descend much or not at all. Multiparas (veterans) may have a modest descent or have significant descent of the baby's head, needing only one or two contractions to complete delivery once the urge is felt.

Q. *How do I know when to push?*

A. The pressure of your baby's head causes a reflex, a bearing-down sensation. This is involuntary and does not have to be learned. This urge is strongest during a contraction. If you have an epidural, you may not feel the urge to push. The monitor tracing may alert your nurse or an exam may reveal full dilation. If you are a multipara or occasionally a primipara, you may be able to push effectively with coaching. If you cannot push effectively, you will "labor down," or let the uterus push the head down through the birth canal while your dose of anesthetic is lowered just enough to allow you to feel the urge to push but not experience pain.

Q. *How do I push?*

A. Wait until you feel the contraction building up and take a slow, deep breath and exhale; then take a deep breath, hold it, and bear down as if you were straining during a bowel movement. Have your coach count slowly to ten, exhale, then inhale rapidly and deeply, hold it, and push to ten again. You will be able to push three times during a contraction. While you are pushing, traditionally you will be lying down with your bed raised at a 30-degree angle. You will put your chin on your chest and pull and hold onto the insides of your knees.

Q. *I heard that there are other pushing positions that are more natural and effective than pushing on my back. Is this true?*

A. Other positions may be used. Some groups believe that pushing in other positions will affect the second stage of labor in a positive way—quicker delivery time and less failure to descend, leading to a decrease in the C-section rate. Studies, however, have not shown such an advantage. But if you would feel more comfortable pushing on your side, in a birthing chair in the knee-chest position, or squatting, go ahead and try it as long as you are comfortable and pushing effectively. There is one complication to pushing for prolonged periods in these positions. A peroneal neuropathy can develop, causing foot drop.

Q. *Do I have to do controlled pushes?*

A. No. If you like, you can bear down and push with urge for as long or as short as you want. However, studies have shown that the time to delivery using this urge-to-push method will prolong your second stage and time of delivery.

Q. *Will I urinate, pass gas, and have a bowel movement when I push?*

A. Yes. If you don't have an epidural and therefore a Foley catheter in your bladder, most women will leak urine at last once while pushing. Some women will spray their urine while pushing if they have a full bladder. If you have not had a bowel movement before labor, you have a great chance of having one during the pushing phase. Don't hold back or be embarrassed. Remember, you do have rectal pressure and you are supposed to push like you are constipated and are trying to have a bowel movement. Your nurses and doctors have seen it, smelled it, and cleaned it up hundreds of times before you and will hundreds of times in the future.

Q. *How long is the second stage of labor?*

A. The average time in primiparas (women giving birth for the first time) is 1 hour, but may be anywhere from 5 minutes to more than 2 hours. The average time in multiparas is 20 minutes, with a range of 1 minute (one push) to 1 hour. The length of time depends on the size of your baby, the size of your pelvis, the position of the baby's head, the quality of your contractions, and the quality of your pushing efforts.

Q. *What is a prolonged second stage of labor?*

A. A prolonged second stage of labor for a primipara is over 2 hours without an epidural and over 3 hours of pushing with an epidural. If you are a multipara, then it's over 1 hour without an epidural and over 2 hours with an epidural.

Q. *Can I push longer if I have the energy?*

A. Yes. Some moms can push for over 3 hours and complete delivery, although it's not too commonplace. You will be allowed to push as long as your baby tolerates this stage and you are making progress.

Q. *What happens if I have a prolonged second stage of labor?*

A. If you still have the energy and you are still making progress and your baby is still tolerating labor and the second stage, you will continue to push. If your pushing efforts are waning in strength, your doctor may suggest the use of a vacuum or forceps to complete the delivery of your baby if the baby's head is low enough in the birth canal. If your baby's head is still high and your pushing efforts are ineffective or have greatly diminished in strength, you will have a cesarean section.

Q. *What is a vacuum extractor?*

A. This is a device that looks like an ice-cream cone and is made of Silastic, a soft, bendable plastic. This device is placed on the crown (back part of the skull that is seen with crowning) of the fetal head and remains attached by applying variable degrees of suction. The purpose of the vacuum is to hold station. For example, in a prolonged second stage, the fetal head may come down the birth canal during a contraction only to rise back up (suck back up) into the vagina as the uterus relaxes. The vacuum will maintain the lowest point of descent of the fetal head, allowing the next contraction and pushing effort to advance your baby down the canal to delivery. The vacuum can also be used if the baby's head is stuck looking sideways (transverse) or up (posterior). The vacuum will gently rotate or assist in the delivery of the head. A vacuum may also be used to help deliver your baby's head if you are exhausted and after an hour or two (or three?) you just don't have the power to complete the delivery. Vacuums are sometimes used to quickly deliver your baby if the baby's heartbeat pattern looks nonreassuring to your doctor and a quick delivery may be in the best interest of your baby's health. Almost all doctors will use the vacuum exclusively.

Q. *What are the alternatives to using a vacuum?*

A. Pushing longer and harder or having a cesarean section.

Q. *What are the risks of using a vacuum for my delivery?*

A. The greatest complication is failure to deliver and the need for a C-section. Risks to the baby are minimal, rare, and self-limiting. The most common risk to the baby is a bruise where the cup was placed. The most common risk to the mom is an episiotomy or vaginal lacerations and tears with or without an episiotomy. But this is to be expected, since the vaginal tissues have been swollen from hours of pushing and the fetal head is just a bit too big to exit. This edema will allow the tissue to tear easily with stretching, which will be stretched even more by this bigger head. I believe that delivery by vacuum extraction is safe when used appropriately. My first child was born as a vacuum-assisted delivery.

Q. *How long will it take to deliver my baby with the vacuum?*

A. Not more than three contractions, because if you haven't delivered by then, you won't. Many times delivery is complete with one assisted push.

Q. *What is crowning?*

A. Crowning occurs when the back of your baby's head, called the crown (for your prince or princess), opens your vagina and stays there so you can see it even between contractions. If you do not have an epidural, you will feel an unpleasant burning sensation as your vagina is being stretched. Your perineum will bulge out, stretching the skin and lengthening the distance between the bottom of your vagina and your anus. The skin in this area will thin out and become increasingly taut and shiny. Your rectal opening will also enlarge quite a bit because it, too, will be stretched by the descent of your baby's head. You may develop one or more hemorrhoids as well.

Q. *How long will crowning last until my baby delivers?*

A. The time can be highly variable and depends on:

- Parity (primiparas take longer to deliver than multiparas)
- Elasticity and size of vaginal opening
- Size of the baby's head
- Spontaneous tears (if your vagina and perineum tear quickly, the baby will deliver quickly)
- Episiotomy (used to hasten delivery of the baby if the baby does not tolerate labor or maternal exhaustion occurs)

Once crowning occurs, you may push for an additional 30 to 60 minutes to stretch out your vagina and perineum if spontaneous tearing does not occur.

Q. *What happens after the baby's head crowns?*

A. As the baby descends farther down the birth canal, the perineum and vagina will distend and thin out even more. Many women without an epidural stop pushing effectively because the burning feeling from the vaginal and perineal stretching is so intense, especially if this is a first delivery. Your vulva and perineum will be washed by the nurse. Your legs will be held by yourself or by your labor coaches or placed in stirrups. Your doctor will be gowned and gloved, and a sterile sheet will be placed under your bottom. During crowning, you must listen to your birth attendant and stop pushing by exhaling to allow the perineum to stretch gradually. You will push and relax until the baby's head has been delivered. During the delivery of the baby's head, your doctor will be pressing against the perineum with his or her hand. This is done to support the tissues of the perineum, protecting them against tearing. Once the baby's head is delivered, you will be asked to stop pushing again. The baby's mouth will then be suctioned and you will then be coached on pushing and not pushing until the shoulders are slowly delivered. The delivery of the shoulders can also cause tears and lacerations of the vagina. The perineum will once again be supported. Remember to inform your physician of your desires and continue to work as a team throughout the delivery process.

Q. *What is an episiotomy?*

A. There are two types of episiotomies, midline and mediolateral. Almost all episiotomies in the United States are midlines. An episiotomy is an incision of the vagina and perineum (the area between the bottom of the vagina and the top of the rectum) and the muscles underlying this area.

If an episiotomy is necessary, a huge snip does not have to be performed. Sometimes all that is required is a ¼- to ½-inch cut of the perineum and vagina and, if necessary, extending the incision superficially into the mucosa (skin) of the vagina. Sometimes the area of the hymenal ring just inside your vagina will not stretch, and after this superficial area is cut on the posterior part of the vagina, your baby's head will advance to crowning.

Q. *When is the episiotomy performed?*

A. An episiotomy is performed if necessary. If a vacuum delivery is required and the vagina and perineum have not been stretched by the head crowning, an episiotomy will be done. If the baby is no longer tolerating labor (even though the head is crowning) and the delivery is not imminent without an episiotomy, one should be performed. If the head has been delivered but the shoulders are stuck (shoulder dystocia), an episiotomy will be performed to allow room for delivery. If the baby's head has been crowning for a long time and the mother is exhausted, an episiotomy may be performed.

Q. *How is it performed?*

A. A pair of curved scissors is used to make the incision. The actual cut with the scissors does not have to be long or deep. A very shallow skin incision can be performed to allow the vagina and perineum to tear naturally if time of delivery is not essential. This may protect you from deep lacerations.

Q. *Is there much bleeding from the episiotomy?*

A. The blood loss is minimal when performed at the proper time, as outlined above.

Q. *Is anesthesia used?*

A. Yes, three different types may be employed. If an epidural is in place, this will be more than adequate to numb the area. Local anesthesia or a pudendal nerve block could be used with an agent such as lidocaine. Some women do not want any anesthesia injected into their body and prefer to be cut when the skin is stretched and the head puts pressure on the skin, causing the skin to be numb. This is called a pressure episiotomy. It still hurts.

Q. *What is local anesthesia?*

A. This is an injection of lidocaine, a local anesthetic. Using a thin needle, this fluid will be injected just under the skin, numbing the nerves in that area. A small pinprick and a burning sensation will be felt during administration of the drug.

Q. *What is the purpose of an episiotomy?*

A. It permits an easier and quicker delivery of your baby when indicated.

Q. *Are there disadvantages to an episiotomy?*

A. The risk of tears into the rectal sphincter and into the rectum is more likely if a standard episiotomy is performed.

Q. *When is the repair of an episiotomy or vaginal lacerations performed?*

A. After the placenta is expelled and the uterus contracts, the doctor will check your cervix and vagina for lacerations and repair these, if necessary. The episiotomy site will then be tested for numbness. Additional anesthesia will be supplied as needed before the repair is begun.

Q. *How long does the repair take?*

A. It will take about 10 minutes for the doctor to sew up the episiotomy site. If the tears are extensive, however, it may take an hour.

Q. *Is there really an extra stitch for the husband?*

A. For the most part, no. The vagina, perineum, and muscles will be sewn back together. Kegel exercises will restore the muscle tone in your vagina. However, if the patient felt that her vagina was loose after a previous vaginal delivery, an extra stitch or two may help, depending on the first episiotomy repair or first repair after a natural tear. Occasionally, a patient will ask that the repair be made so that the vagina is not as tight as before delivery. This can be done as well.

Q. *Is an episiotomy necessary?*

A. This debate has been going on since episiotomies became a commonplace practice in the United States in 1945. It is not necessary in all situations and should not be a routine procedure in all deliveries. Episiotomies are more commonly performed by doctors than nurse-midwives. The episiotomy rate for some physicians may be as high as 100 percent. The midwife rate is as low as 15 percent. The episiotomy rate in the Netherlands is only 7 percent. Why is there such a discrepancy in the episiotomy rates? Part of the answer lies in training—the training of the doctor and of the patient. Part of the answer may be the larger babies born under the care of physicians in the United States. If an episiotomy is not performed, at least 75 percent of the time the vagina will tear and require suture repair, according to the midwife literature. They have a better rate than I do. Most physicians will try not to perform an episiotomy; a no-episiotomy, no-tear birth is a welcome end to labor, but not a common event in first-time moms.

Q. *Does third-trimester perineal massage help avoid perineal/vaginal tears or an episiotomy?*

A. In one study, the practice of perineal self-massage decreased the rate of nonsignificant tears by 6 percent in first-time births and had no effect in subsequent births.

Q. *Can my position during delivery affect the likelihood of vaginal tears?*

A. No. You are just as likely to tear if you are lying back down, squatting, standing, using a balance ball, or lying on your side.

Q. *Will perineal massage and vaginal stretching during the second (pushing) stage increase my chance of delivering with an intact perineum?*

A. No. There is the same risk of vaginal and perineal tears. In fact, perineal massage did not decrease the risk of pain, future pain with intercourse, or urinary or fecal incontinence. This practice may also cause tearing, abrasions, and discomfort, especially in you first-time moms with swollen (edematous) tissues.

Q. *What are the degrees of vaginal/perineal tears or lacerations?*

A. There are four degrees of tearing:

- First-degree tear. The tear is through the skin of the vagina and or perineum and or labia and or clitoris.
- Second-degree tear. The tear extends through the skin of the vagina and perineum and into the different muscles of the vagina and perineum down to the capsule of the anal sphincter (the muscle around the anus that allows you to control your ability to hold flatus or stool).
- Third-degree tear. The tear extends down to and tears the capsule and muscle of the anal sphincter.

- Fourth-degree tear. The tear extends through the vaginal and perineal skin, muscle, anal sphincter capsule and muscle and through the rectal mucosa.

There can also be combinations of all four types of tears occurring all at once after a delivery. The extent of the tears depends on the size and elasticity of the vaginal mucosa and muscles, the length of the perineum, presence of tissue edema, episiotomy and size of episiotomy, the size of the baby, controlled delivery versus uncontrolled pushing after crowning, protection of the perineum with delivery versus none, instrumental delivery, and first-time mom versus experienced mom. Your vagina might have one tear or multiple tears of different degrees in different locations around your vagina and perineum.

Q. *Can I use a mirror to see my baby when I deliver?*

A. Yes. Most LDRs (labor, delivery, and recovery rooms) are equipped with mirrors that can be set up so you can view the delivery of your baby. Most of the time, however, you will be so intent on pushing your baby out that you forget about looking and have your eyes closed while pushing. You may at least see your baby crowning.

Q. *What happens once the baby's head is delivered?*

A. The doctor will check for any loops of cord wrapped around the baby's neck and uncoil them. A bulb syringe will then be placed in the baby's mouth and nostrils to remove excess mucus and amniotic fluid. Gentle traction will be placed on the baby's head and you will be asked to push. The baby's shoulders will rotate and will be eased out one at a time. The rest of the baby follows quickly. The baby's nose and mouth will be cleared once again.

Q. *Where does my baby go after it is born?*

A. I place the baby on the new mother's (now flatter) abdomen. Don't be afraid to touch your baby or cuddle and hug him or her.

Q. *Can I breast-feed my baby right after he or she is born?*

A. As long as everything has progressed normally, you can try. Most babies aren't that hungry right after their trip down the birth canal; they'd rather get warm and breathe. Some babies will start nursing about 20 to 30 minutes after birth, and others may not be interested for hours.

Q. *When does the baby start crying?*

A. Your baby will start crying within 1 minute after birth. Crying expands your baby's lungs and begins the normal process of breathing. This also shifts the circulation from fetal to newborn.

Q. *Who clamps and cuts the cord?*

A. Ask your doctor about this one. After a normal delivery, many doctors will let your mate (or significant other) clamp and cut the cord. Ask the nurse to take the photographs.

Q. *I heard that it is better to wait until the cord stops beating before clamping the cord. Is that true?*

A. If the fetus was anemic (extremely rare) and requires as much blood as possible, then delaying the clamping of the cord might be necessary. The baby, however, must be held below the level of your vagina to accomplish this. With most deliveries, there is no advantage in delaying clamping the cord.

Q. *What is the Apgar score?*

A. The Apgar score is physical evaluation of the newborn. It is used to rate the condition of your baby's health after undergoing the stress of labor. The Apgar score was devised by Dr. Virginia Apgar, an obstetrical anesthesiologist, in 1958. The ratings are given at 1 and 5 minutes. The best score is a 10, but this is rare; usually, the highest score given will be a 9—no one is perfect. Most babies have a score of from 7 to 9 at 1 and 5 minutes. A low score (less than 5) at 1 minute indicates a depressed baby who may require some sort of resuscitation. A low score (less than 5) at 5 minutes may be associated with an increased risk of neurological problems later in life.

Q. *Who gives the Apgar score?*

A. With a normal delivery or during a cesarean section, the nurse assigns the Apgar score.

Q. *What else does the nurse do with my baby in the delivery room?*

A. She or he will take footprints of your baby and place them on the birth certificate (along with your fingerprints), place an identification bracelet around the ankle and wrist (and an identical one on your wrist), give your baby an injection of vitamin K, and place an antibiotic ointment in the eyes.

Q. *Why does my baby need an injection of vitamin K?*

A. Newborns do not have an adequate supply of vitamin K, which is necessary for blood clotting.

Q. *Why is antibiotic ointment placed in my baby's eyes?*

A. An antibiotic (erythromycin) ointment is administered to prevent an eye infection from gonorrhea or chlamydia transmitted from the mother. Silver nitrate was used in the past, but it was irritating to the newborn's eyes. The current ointments are not. I know because I put them in my own eyes. Most states require by law that medication be used to prevent these infections.

Q. *When does the placenta come out?*

A. Most often the placenta spontaneously separates after 5 minutes, but up to 25 minutes is not abnormally long. You may notice a gush of blood (1 cup) and another uterine contraction. Your doctor may ask you to push one last time to complete the delivery of the placenta. If you so desire, ask your doctor to show you the placenta.

Q. *What happens if the placenta does not detach spontaneously?*

A. This is a rare event. The doctor will have to manually remove the placenta. A hand is placed in the uterus to shear the placenta off the wall of the uterus. This procedure may be painful but is performed in seconds. If your relaxation breathing does not allow you to manage the pain, ask for a pain reliever, an epidural, or general anesthesia.

Q. *What happens after the placenta is expelled?*

A. There is usually some bleeding and clots of blood following the placenta. Your uterus may not contract right away and bleeding may continue. To contract the uterus, you may try nursing your baby (stimulation of your nipple causes the release of oxytocin), the doctor will firmly and gently massage your uterus, causing it to contract, or the nurse will give you an injection of Pitocin into a muscle or through an IV to cause uterine contractions. Discuss which method your doctor employs. It is important for your uterus to contract to prevent excessive blood loss.

After the delivery of the placenta, you may develop some tremors, or the "postpartum shakes." This is quite normal. Your body has just been through a great deal of exercise. The shakes only last a couple of minutes.

Your doctor will then examine your cervix and vagina for any possible tears and repair them along with the episiotomy, if one was performed. Your nurse will then clean you up and put the labor bed back together. Most hospitals allow family members or friends to wait just outside the labor and delivery area and greet the new family as soon as you desire.

Q. *What is postpartum hemorrhage?*

A. Postpartum hemorrhage is excessive vaginal bleeding after the expulsion of the placenta. The most common cause of postpartum hemorrhage is uterine atony.

Q. *What is uterine atony?*

A. Uterine atony means that the uterus does not want to contract or stay contracted.

A well-contracted uterus does not bleed heavily; one that is flaccid will. The muscular contraction of the uterus is the mechanism by which the uterus controls the bleeding from the placental site.

Q. *How common is uterine atony?*

A. This problem occurs quite frequently. The incidence is about 1 in 20 births.

Q. *Who is at risk for uterine atony?*

A. If you have a pregnancy that causes your uterus to be overdistended, you are at risk. This can be caused by a twin (or greater) pregnancy, polyhydramnios (too much amniotic fluid), or a very large baby. A rapid labor and delivery or a prolonged labor with hours of Pitocin, a prolonged second stage with hours of pushing, and then a forceps, vacuum, or C-section delivery increases your risk for uterine atony. If you have already had four or more children, you are at higher risk as well. The use of magnesium sulfate for preeclampsia can also increase the risk of uterine atony.

Q. *What is the treatment for uterine atony?*

A. The treatment begins with clearing blood clots out of the uterus, uterine massage, and IV Pitocin. If these measures fail, your bladder will be drained with a Foley catheter. A methylergonovine maleate (Methergine) or prostaglandin intramuscular injection may then be used to stimulate uterine contractions. Blood loss may be excessive; blood transfusion is rare, but your postpartum recovery may be complicated by the fatigue of anemia.

Q. *What happens after my delivery?*

A. You will stay in the LDR for about 2 hours. During this time, the nurses will check your blood pressure, pulse, and temperature every 15 minutes. In addition, your fundus will be massaged to ensure that it has contracted, and you will be examined for the quantity of blood flow. If you are hungry, food will be served. Your baby will stay with you for about 2 hours.

Q. *Can my partner give the baby a bath after birth?*

A. Sure. About 2 hours after the birth, your baby will be taken to the nursery for assessment. Your baby will be placed in the warmer for this. After the normal physical exam, your baby will get its first bath by your partner or the nursing staff.

Q. *What is "back labor"?*

A. "Back labor" is so named because the pains of labor are felt most intensely in the back.

Q. *Why do some women experience back labor?*

A. The intensity of labor pains or where the pains are felt the most depends on the individual and her nervous system. Many individuals believe that back labor occurs when the baby's head is in the occiput posterior, or face-up, position. I have not found this to be the case in my own practice, and just by statistics, this presentation occurs in only 1 in 200 deliveries.

Q. *Is labor more common during a full moon?*

A. Although both doctors and patients seem to believe that the moon influences the onset of labor, this is not so. This myth was dispelled by a Dr. Witter, who demonstrated through an elaborate study that the full moon had no influence on the number of deliveries or on women in active labor (in Baltimore, at least).

Q. *Are more babies born in the middle of the night?*

A. Fortunately for your doctor and possibly you, no. The percentage of babies born throughout the day is about equal.

Q. *When is the safest time of day to have my baby?*

A. The safest time to deliver is during the day. There is an increased risk of minor and major complications when deliveries occur between 7 P.M. and 12 A.M. and a slightly higher complication rate between 1 A.M. and 6 A.M.

ANALGESICS AND ANESTHESIA FOR LABOR AND DELIVERY

Q. *I am in labor and I am in pain.*
Will walking reduce my need for
analgesia (pain relief medicine/epidural)?

A. No. The pain will be the same in intensity. In fact, sitting, squatting, or using a balance ball will not lessen the need for pain relief.

Q. *Will lying in a hot tub with jets*
decrease my need for analgesia?

A. No. It might delay your request for pain meds/epidural, but the pain will be just as intense.

Q. *If I need relief from the pain of labor,*
what is available?

A. Sedatives, narcotics, tranquilizers, epidural, or spinal anesthesia may be given to provide pain relief during labor. You must ask for something for pain relief if you want it.

Q. *When would my doctor give me a sedative?*

A. Sedatives, such as a sleeping pill, are given in the latent phase of labor if you cannot rest when the contractions are still irregular.

Q. *What are the effects on me?*

A. The sedative should make you drowsy and allow you to sleep until the contractions become more regular and forceful. If you are in labor, a sedative will not slow it down.

Q. *What are the effects on the fetus?*

A. The same as on you, drowsiness and sleep. Sedatives are usually only given, if needed, in the latent phase of first pregnancies, so the effects of the drug on the fetus have worn off long before delivery.

Q. *When are narcotics given?*

A. Narcotics are given in the late part of the latent phase and during the active phase.

Q. *How effective are narcotics in relieving pain?*

A. With minimal to moderate pain in early labor, relief is attained up to 50 percent of the time. Narcotics also reduce the anxiety you may experience from the pain of labor.

Q. *How are narcotics administered?*

A. Narcotics are given by either intramuscular injection or through an intravenous line.

Q. *Will narcotic medication slow my labor?*

A. No. In fact, your labor may be shortened by the medicine.

Q. *Which narcotics may be used?*

A. Meperidine (Demerol) is one of the most common drugs used. Others are nalbuphine hydrochloride (Nubain) and butorphanol tartrate (Stadol).

Q. *How fast does Stadol or Demerol work, and how long do the effects last?*

A. If given through your IV, you will start to feel the effects within 1 minute. Maximal pain relief will occur in 5 minutes and last for about 1 to 2 hours, depending on the dose given. If an intramuscular injection is given, pain relief will begin in about 10 minutes, have maximal effect in 45 minutes, and last from 2 to 3 hours, again depending on the drug and dose administered.

Q. *What are the side effects of narcotic medication on me?*

A. Drowsiness, nausea and vomiting, and respiratory depression may occur.

Q. *Can I have a medicine to prevent these side effects?*

A. Yes. As a matter of fact, many doctors give a tranquilizer (promethazine hydrochloride, trade name Phenergan; or hydroxyzine pamoate, trade name Vistaril) with the narcotic to prevent the nausea and vomiting. In addition, the tranquilizer will add to the effects of the narcotic. This means that less of the narcotic will be given to effect the same degree of pain relief. But it is a tranquilizer, so you will be even drowsier when you take this medicine. Your labor experience will be lost in a fog of narcosis.

Q. *What are the side effects on the fetus?*

A. The narcotic will enter the fetal circulation in 1 to 5 minutes, depending on the route of administration. The side effects are the same as above but last longer in the fetus. Your doctor will not administer a narcotic close to delivery to avoid respiratory depression of your baby at birth. If this happens, however, a narcotic antagonist may be given to the baby to reverse the effects.

Q. *Are there any long-term effects on my baby?*

A. There are no neurological or developmental effects on the baby.

Q. *What is an epidural?*

A. It is an injection of a local anesthetic through your back and in between the segments of your bony spine into the epidural space, a potential space between the dura (the covering membrane of the spinal cord and fluid) and the surrounding tissues.

Q. *What is a one-shot epidural?*

A. A one-shot epidural is just that: one dose of anesthetic is injected through the epidural needle and then the needle is removed. This used to be the most common form of epidural administered. Now it is rarely performed for labor anesthesia; instead, a catheter (tube) is usually placed.

Q. *What is a continuous low-dose epidural?*

A. A continuous low-dose epidural constantly injects a low dose of an anesthetic agent. After the anesthesiologist finds the epidural space with the needle, a catheter is placed through the needle into the epidural space, and the needle is removed. A bolus dose of anesthetic can first be administered to ensure pain relief within 10 to 20 minutes. The catheter is then hooked up to a pump that will supply a predetermined constant infusion of anesthetic.

Q. *What are the advantages of a continuous low-dose epidural?*

A. The advantages are:

- The continuous epidural provides constant pain relief— no need to worry about the anesthetic completely wearing off before the anesthesiologist reinjects you.
- Low dose of medicine means fewer side effects.
- Low dose of anesthetic should not block motor function to your lower extremities.
- The dose may be readjusted easily to afford more or less pain relief during the different stages of labor.
- Anesthetic may be turned off at any time, with the return of sensation within 20 to 30 minutes.

Q. *What is a light epidural?*

A. The light epidural contains a narcotic, such as fentanyl, Demerol, or morphine, along with the anesthetic agent. The addition of the narcotic enables the anesthesiologist to give you less anesthetic, so you are less numb, have better control over your lower extremities, and can push more effectively because you are able to experience the pressure and bearing-down sensations without the accompanying pain.

Q. *Who gives it?*

A. It is administered by the anesthesiologist.

Q. *How does it work?*

A. The nerves leaving and entering the spinal column are bathed in the local anesthetic and are numbed.

Q. *What special preparations are needed before placement?*

A. You will need an IV for hydration. A blood pressure cuff will be placed on your arm to monitor your blood pressure at short intervals after the epidural is activated.

Q. *Should I get an epidural or pain medication during labor?*

A. If you are in intolerable pain, sure. Many women prefer to go through labor without the assistance of a pain reliever. If you can, great. But even if you were not planning to have an epidural, keep an open mind about getting one if the pain is unbearable. Remember, your doctor and labor nurses are never in pain during your labor; they are there to help.

Q. *When can I ask for an epidural?*

A. As soon as you feel that the pain is unbearable. This usually occurs during transition. Some women who had pain with prior pregnancies will request an epidural in early labor before the pain becomes too intense. An epidural at this time may slow labor considerably, widening the interval between contractions. Pitocin may be used in this situation to enhance labor.

Studies have now shown that there is no increase in the rate of cesarean sections if an epidural is placed in early labor (2 to 3 centimeters dilated). Some women will ask and receive their epidural soon after induction of labor with Pitocin.

Q. *How soon will I have pain relief?*

A. Usually in about 20 minutes. First, the anesthesiologist will give you a small test dose of the drug and observe for side effects. If none occur after 10 minutes, a full dose will be given. Its effects will be appreciated in 10 minutes.

Q. *What will I feel?*

A. You will feel no more pain from uterine contractions; in fact, you will not even feel them. You will be numb from the top of your uterus to the tips of your toes! You will not feel the urge to urinate either so you will have a Foley catheter placed to drain urine from your bladder.

Q. *How long does the anesthesia last?*

A. Continuous low-dose epidural is the standard in the United States. The anesthetic lasts until you have delivered.

Q. *What are the advantages?*

A. Clearly, the main advantage is pain relief. Another plus occurs in the previously agitated woman in intense pain and slow progress in labor; the relief of pain may quicken cervical dilation and relax the muscles of the pelvic floor, hastening the end of the first stage of labor. Also, with the catheter in place, the anesthesiologist can selectively provide pain relief to the perineum during the second stage of labor or administer anesthesia for a cesarean section if one becomes necessary.

Q. *In what circumstances should an epidural not be placed?*

A. If there is heavy vaginal bleeding, an infection near the injection site, selected previous back surgeries, selected neurological diseases, a low platelet count, or certain blood disorders, an epidural should not be placed.

Q. *What complications may occur?*

A. The most common complication is an unwanted motor blockade along with the desired sensory blockade. If your motor nerves are numb, you will experience "dead legs." You will temporarily not be able to move your legs. Worse, however, is the fact that you could be completely dilated and yet not feel the urge to push for potentially more than 2 hours. To prevent this from occurring, move both legs every 15 minutes. If you start losing strength in one of your legs, have the nurse call the anesthesiologist to readjust your dose. Sometimes after the anesthetic is administered, you can experience a temporary decrease in your blood pressure. This hypotension could cause no symptoms or could cause nausea and dizziness and a transient drop in your baby's heart rate. The blood pressure changes are easily reversed with more IV fluids, oxygen, and medicine.

The following complications may occur, though they are extremely rare: The anesthetic may be ineffective. A spinal anesthetic may be inadvertently administered, leading to complications of spinal anesthesia. Hypotension (low blood pressure) may be induced. Even rarer, convulsions can occur if the local anesthetic is injected into a blood vessel instead of into the epidural space.

Q. *What are the effects on the baby?*

A. With the properly selected anesthetic agent, there is minimal transfer of drug to the fetus, since the drug is broken down by plasma in your bloodstream and the placenta.

Q. *Will an epidural slow down my labor?*

A. Sometimes, and sometimes it might speed it up. If your contractions space out, then you will receive Pitocin to augment your labor. You won't feel it now that you have an epidural. If you were in labor and not progressing and barely tolerating the pain of contractions, you and your cervix will relax after the epidural is placed, and you may dilate more rapidly.

Q. *What is spinal anesthesia?*

A. This is anesthesia provided by injecting the anesthetic agent into the spinal cord.

Q. *How is it given?*

A. The same way as with the epidural, only the needle punctures the dura and the drug bathes and numbs the nerves in the spinal column.

Q. *What are the effects of spinal anesthesia?*

A. Effects include complete loss of sensation and muscle function in the area the nerves anesthetized supply.

Q. *When is it given?*

A. Spinal anesthesia is the preferred anesthesia for an elective cesarean section. It may also be used for an unplanned nonemergency cesarean section in a mom who did not have an epidural during labor.

Q. *What are the possible complications*
   of a spinal anesthesia?

A. The most notorious complication is a spinal headache, which actually occurs in less than 1 percent of patients. As with an epidural, low blood pressure and a total spinal anesthesia may rarely occur. Meningitis is an extremely rare complication.

Q. *What is the treatment for a spinal headache?*

A. Mild headaches are treated with ibuprophen, caffeine, extra fluids, and lying down on your back. If your headache persists and becomes more painful, your anesthesiologist will assess you for treatment with a "blood patch." Blood will be taken from your arm and placed around the hole that was previously created in the dura (the membrane surrounding the spinal cord and fluid). Treatment with the blood patch is 75 percent effective.

MECONIUM

Q. *What is meconium?*

A. Meconium is the dark green feces of the fetus (or newborn). If the fetus has a bowel movement while in your uterus, the fluid may be yellowish, light green, or dark green, depending on the amount of meconium passed and the amount of amniotic fluid present. Similarly, the consistency of the meconium-stained fluid may be watery or like pea soup.

Q. *Why does the baby pass meconium?*

A. Your fetus may pass meconium as a response to the compression of his or her umbilical cord or to a decrease in oxygen supply. Or it may be a normal bodily function of the mature fetus.

Q. *How common is meconium?*

A. Meconium-stained amniotic fluid may be seen in up to 20 percent of pregnancies at term and up to 40 percent at 42 weeks.

Q. *What is the significance of meconium?*

A. Meconium by itself rarely indicates that your fetus is having a problem. If there is meconium present in the amniotic fluid and your fetus appears to tolerate labor well, the baby will do just fine. If there is thick meconium-stained fluid and the fetus exhibits signs of not tolerating contractions during labor, then there is a greater chance that your baby may be depressed at birth and have a lower Apgar score. One other thing to look for is an unsuspected breech presentation; meconium passage is a frequent occurrence in breech births.

Q. *What is amnioinfusion?*

A. Amnioinfusion is the placement of a normal saline (salt) solution into your uterus through the intrauterine pressure catheter. This procedure is done in laboring patients.

Q. *Why might I have an amnioinfusion*
performed on me?

A. Amnioinfusions may be performed during the following scenarios:

- *Thick meconium.* Adding clear fluid to an amniotic cavity with thick meconium will first dilute the meconium, then wash the meconium out. This will decrease the potential complications of meconium aspiration syndrome (MAS) to your newborn, and it has been shown that amnioinfusion in this situation has decreased the likelihood of cesarean sections and low Apgar scores (the index used to evaluate the condition of a newborn).

- *Oligohydramnios.* Decreased amniotic fluid may occur in preterm laboring patients, in postterm laboring patients, and in IUGR pregnancies. When there is decreased amniotic fluid, there is more of a chance of having cord compression during a contraction. This may be seen on the fetal heart monitor as variable or late decelerations, a potentially ominous sign. Amnioinfusion has been shown to reverse these patterns and decrease the need for an operative intervention.
- *Fetal distress.* As stated above, in certain situations the use of amnioinfusion may reverse a potentially life-threatening situation without the need of cesarean section.

Q. *Is amnioinfusion safe?*

A. When the proper guidelines are follwed, amnioinfusion appears to be quite safe. The infused salt solution is quite similar to the salts found in your amniotic fluid. Overinfusion should not be a problem because the medical staff will be watching the pressure catheter during the infusion.

Q. *What does the doctor do if I have meconium during labor?*

A. Your doctor will use internal fetal monitors to more closely monitor the heart rate pattern of your fetus during and in between contractions. In addition, amnioinfusion can be performed to flush out existing meconium. After the delivery of your baby's head, your doctor will carefully suction out any meconium in your baby's nose, mouth, and throat and will continue to do so as the body is being delivered. If the meconium is thick, your doctor will cut the umbilical cord, take your baby to the warmer, and, using a laryngoscope, look at your baby's vocal cords and suction out the trachea for any remaining meconium. This is done to prevent meconium aspiration syndrome.

Q. *What is meconium aspiration syndrome (MAS)?*

A. MAS is a condition due to meconium in the lungs. It causes inflammation of the lungs and breathing problems for the newborn. Most cases of MAS occur before the baby is born, but the management discussed previously will lessen the severity of this syndrome greatly.

INDUCTION OF LABOR

Q. *What is induction of labor?*

A. Induction of labor is the process of beginning labor through artificial means. This should only be accomplished by your doctor.

Q. *What is amniotomy?*

A. Amniotomy is the artificial rupture of your chorioamniotic membranes by your doctor. This is usually performed by a plastic device called an *amnihook*, which looks like a crochet needle. It is also called "breaking your water."

Q. *Why would I have an amniotomy?*

A. An amniotomy may be performed for an induction of labor, as part of an augmentation of labor, or routinely by some doctors during the active phase of labor to shorten that phase of labor, to apply a fetal scalp electrode if external monitoring is not accurate enough and to place an intrauterine pressure catheter (IUPC) if necessary.

Q. *What are the disadvantages of routine amniotomy?*

A. There may be an increased incidence of mild to moderate variable decelerations after artificial rupture of membranes, but these changes are not severe enough to cause an increased chance of cesarean section or low Apgar scores. There is no increased incidence of infection in you or your baby unless, of course, your labor lasts much longer than 18 hours after amniotomy. Labor contractions may be more painful following amniotomy. Very rarely, the umbilical cord can prolapse through the cervix, which would require an immediate cesarean section.

Q. *What are the advantages of routine amniotomy?*

A. Elective amniotomy in the active phase will shorten your active phase significantly. In one study, the difference was 6 hours with unruptured membranes versus 4½ hours with amniotomy! Cesarean section rates will be the same, but there is less need for Pitocin administration in the artificially ruptured laboring patient to accomplish a vaginal delivery.

Q. *Why would I have an induction of labor?*

A. Induction of labor is necessary in a variety of conditions. The situations prompting an induction of labor may be due to either a maternal medical condition or a fetal indication:

- Mild preeclampsia at term or severe preeclampsia near term
- Postterm pregnancy: your pregnancy has gone 2 or more weeks past your due date
- Rh disease worsening at or near term
- FGR near term
- Decreased fetal movement with a nonreactive nonstress test near term
- Gestational diabetes or diabetes mellitus near term
- Oligohydramnios (decreased amniotic fluid) with fetal heart rate changes near term
- Macrosomia: Your baby is estimated to be very large and delivery may be complicated. Actually, the induction would be performed before the baby becomes large. Therefore, the indication would really be for suspected impending macrosomia.

Q. *What about an elective induction of labor?*

A. An induction may be performed when there is a previous history of rapid labor (less than 4 hours) and your cervix is already dilated to more than 3 centimeters or if false labor is bothersome enough to cause sleeplessness.

A particular date close to term might also be chosen if the cervix is ripe.

Elective induction of labor is often chosen by the mom because she is uncomfortable. Inductions are performed for convenience as well, such as the husband's work schedule or babysitting problems. The date can be chosen just as a date is chosen for a C-section. Inductions can be performed up to 2 weeks before your due date if your cervix is ripe. The choice of this procedure for these reasons, however, should be discussed with your doctor.

Q. *What are the advantages of an induction of labor?*

A. If you have a history of rapid labor, your induction-to-delivery time may be shortened considerably. The induction is usually begun in the morning, and therefore a good night's sleep before labor begins can be anticipated. The expectant mother will be told to fast overnight so the possibility of vomiting food will be eliminated. There will be a full complement of nurses, operating crew, and anesthesiologists present during a daytime induction in case a problem arises. Prior arrangements with an anesthesiologist may be made for a placement of an epidural catheter in early labor before contractions become painful, if you desire. Prior arrangements can also be made regarding your partner's schedule and care for your other children.

Q. *What are the potential complications of induction of labor?*

A. Before the advent of prostaglandins, the most common complication was failure to dilate and a resultant cesarean section, which occurred in about 50 percent of cases. The induction of labor in unripe cervixes with prostaglandins (Cervidil [dinoprostone] or misoprostol) has a success rate of more than 70 percent. Now the most common complication of induction is the length of labor; this may be a whole-day affair with an unripe cervix. But remember, the ripening process is not an uncomfortable period of time. Abnormal uterine contractions with Cervidil occur in less than 5 percent of inductions and in less than 4 percent of inductions with Pitocin. Some physicians will place an IUPC to monitor the strength of your contractions, requiring you to stay in bed throughout the induction.

If your baby's head is not engaged and an amniotomy is performed, a prolapsed umbilical cord could rarely occur. If your pregnancy is not close to term, but your medical condition or your baby's condition necessitates an induction, your baby may be born with immature lungs, leading to respiratory complications at birth.

Q. *How will I have my induction of labor with Pitocin?*

A. The prerequisite for a Pitocin induction is a ripe cervix: one that is about 50 percent effaced, soft, and dilated to 2 to 3 centimeters, with the head down and not floating. You will present to L&D in the morning, around 7:30 P.M. Have a light breakfast that morning. After being admitted, an NST will be performed. Once the NST is reactive, you will have an IV started. Antibiotics will be started if you are GBS positive. The Pitocin will be started at a low dose and progressively increased as needed throughout labor. Have a consult with the anesthesiologist now when you are not in pain about placement of an epidural if you desire one. The epidural can be placed and activated at any time. Artificial rupture of membranes may occur soon after admission or when desired by your doctor. Discuss these options with your physician before your induction. After your epidural placement, you may have a Foley catheter placed to drain your bladder. An

IUPC may be placed to monitor the strength of your contractions because you will not be able to feel their intensity. The desired goal of an elective or indicated induction is a safe labor that can be accomplished in a timely manner.

Pitocin will be administered through an IV line with an infusion pump. The Pitocin is given at a low dose initially and gradually increased every 30 minutes if necessary. The peak action of Pitocin takes 20 minutes, and in many cases the dose may be increased several times, which may mean hours before you feel any discomfort from the uterine contractions. The effects of Pitocin work much faster with ruptured membranes. The discomfort begins when your cervix thins out, which, as in a natural labor, may take a few hours after your contractions begin (the latent phase). Once you have regular and strong contractions, your body may once again take over and the amount of Pitocin infused may be decreased or stopped.

Q. *How long will an elective induction using Pitocin take before I have my baby?*

A. The answer depends on many variables: number of deliveries, ripeness of cervix, size of mom and baby, and pushing abilities. The goal is to have you safely deliver within 12 to 16 hours from admission if this is your first pregnancy and less than that if you have already had kids. Most doctors would not advise an elective induction with Pitocin if they thought that the delivery would take longer than that.

Q. *Can I try an induction without Pitocin?*

A. If your cervix is very ripe, all you may need is amniotomy. The artificial rupture of membranes may release enough natural prostaglandins to begin uterine contractions in 1 to 2 hours. If this does not occur, you may be asked to begin nipple stimulation. Nipple stimulation will cause the release of your own oxytocin, causing you to go into labor. You will gently roll your nipple between your thumb and forefinger or gently caress your nipple with your hand in a back and forth motion until you experience a contraction. You stop stimulation at this point and resume at the end of the contraction. Never stimulate both nipples at the same time; this may cause a prolonged and painful contraction that stops blood flow to your baby.

If the combination of amniotomy and nipple stimulation is successful and you are experiencing regular uterine contractions every 3 minutes, you may stop the nipple stimulation and see if your body has now taken over. Unfortunately, this method does not have a high success rate, and even when it does, it dramatically lengthens the induction-to-delivery interval, which can increase the infection rate and tire out many moms when the second stage occurs in the late evening or early morning hours of the next day.

Q. *How many hours will my labor last if I am induced with Pitocin for an indicated reason?*

A. Length of labor depends on the condition of the cervix (dilation and effacement) at the start of the induction and past labor history. For example, if this is your first pregnancy and your cervix is only 1 centimeter dilated and 50 percent effaced, your first stage of labor could last 12 hours or more. But if this is your third pregnancy and your cervix is dilated to 3 or 4 centimeters and completely effaced, your first stage of labor may be only 1 or 2 hours following onset of regular contractions.

Q. *Are uterine contractions more painful*
if I have an induction of labor
with Pitocin?

A. No. Pitocin will cause your uterus to contract just as hard as if you went into labor spontaneously. In fact, although the uterine contractions will initially register strong on the internal monitors, you will not perceive them as such until your cervix completes its effacement and starts to dilate. Many women who have an arrest of dilation will require Pitocin for augmentation of labor. These moms will complain about the increased intensity of painful uterine contractions or increased frequency of contractions because their contractions were mild and not strong enough to dilate the cervix. In this case, Pitocin can cause more painful, but more effective, contractions.

Q. *What happens if I have an unripe*
cervix and need to be induced?

A. If your cervix is not ready—and there are many cervixes that are not—your doctor will suggest an induction with a prostaglandin. There are two types in use, Cervidil and misoprostol. The choice will be whatever your doctor is more comfortable using. You will be admitted to L&D in the early evening. Have a good lunch and a light dinner before coming to the hospital. The nurses will admit you, take your history and vital signs, and hook you up to the external fetal monitor. An NST will be performed until your baby is reactive. Then the prostaglandin will be placed in the back of your vagina and you will remain in bed for about an hour sitting or lying around to be monitored. After about an hour, you can get up and take a walk or remain in bed. You will stay in the hospital overnight, and your significant other may stay with you, too. The cervical ripening trial with prostaglandins is about 12 hours. Three events may occur during this time:

1. You will go into labor. Get an epidural whenever.
2. Your cervix changes (unripe to ripe). You may not know that you have had a change in your cervix because you do not have to experience contractions for this to happen. You are checked in the morning and now your cervix is 2 to 3 centimeters dilated, soft, and at least 50 percent effaced. You can now proceed with amniotomy and a Pitocin induction and epidural if desired.
3. Your cervix did not change. Your doctor may perform a serial induction, which is letting you rest awhile and then repeating with a new trial of prostaglandins. If your baby looked fine the whole night, your doctor may send you home for a few days, and if you don't go into spontaneous labor, you may need to try the process again.

Q. *How do I know if the cervical ripening will work?*

A. You don't, and neither does your doctor. We know that the success rate with these agents is at least 70 percent.

Q. *What are the complications with prostaglandin use?*

A. The major problem is the potential for very long contractions (over 2 minutes) or contractions that are one after another. Both types of hyperstimulation may cause a decrease of blood flow to the baby. Fortunately, most fetuses tolerate this complication. This may happen up to 5 percent of the time, which is why you are monitored in the hospital.

Q. *What is stripping the membranes?*

A. Your cervix must be dilated for the doctor to perform this maneuver. The doctor's finger is placed through the cervix, circling two to three times between the lower part of your uterus and the baby's head and membranes. This will release prostaglandins that may induce labor over the next few hours. The procedure takes less than 15 seconds, may be mildly to moderately uncomfortable (obviously more uncomfortable than just checking your cervix for dilation), and may cause spotting or bleeding and clotting from the cervix, which will stop. It really doesn't work well. If you are dilated and want to have your baby, be induced in the hospital with Pitocin.

Q. *I heard that there are natural oils that can be placed on the cervix that can put me into labor. There are also natural herbs I can take or massage. What do you think about these methods?*

A. If any of these natural methods worked well, a pharmaceutical company would be marketing them. All medicines used for cervical ripening or induction have gone through the scrutiny and approval of the FDA for effectiveness and safety. Your doctor's ultimate goal is the safety of both of his/her patients—you and your baby. Trust your doctor.

Q. *I understand that I have a medical indication for induction, but I want my baby to pick when the birth will be. Can I?*

A. Once your doctor has explained why an induction is appropriate, you may sign a informed refusal form. I really do not understand the concept that the baby picks the delivery time. Medical science does not know what initiates labor. We do not believe that the baby initiates labor, since anencephalic (no brain) babies and stillborn babies can go into labor spontaneously.

Q. *What is cord blood banking?*

A. Cord blood banking is the storage of your child's umbilical cord blood for stem cells. These stem cells can transform into any type of cell in your body, including the cells in the immune system.

Q. *Should I store my baby's blood?*

A. The stem cells in your baby's cord blood may be used to treat some rare diseases in childhood. These cells may also treat diseases in your other children or you and your husband if the amount of blood collected is sufficient to treat a person heavier than 100 pounds, which often is not the case.

Q. *How is cord blood collected?*

A. Your doctor will easily collect it for you after the cord is clamped and cut.

Q. *What is the cost?*

A. The cost ranges from $1,000 to $2,000 and $100 per year.

Q. *Can I donate my baby's cord blood?*

A. Yes. Cryobanks International is a bank that will accept cord blood donation.

Q. *Does the American College of Obstetricians and Gynecologists endorse the routine use of private cord blood banking?*

A. No, at this time they do not. Stem cells cannot be used to treat your child's inborn errors of metabolism because the stem cells have the same genetic defect. Some subtypes of leukemia have the same chromosomal errors, so pediatric hematologists (blood disorder specialists) won't use umbilical cord blood. The estimated chance that an individual might need to use the cord blood is 1 in 2,700.

Q. *Does the American Academy of Pediatrics endorse the private banking of cord blood?*

A. No. They do not endorse individual banking for family biological insurance. They do endorse the donation of cord blood to a public bank to allow for a greater access to the potential of stem cells.

Q. *What is a water birth?*

A. A water birth involves laboring and even delivery in a bathtub or hot tub.

Q. *Is a water birth safe?*

A. Water births in a hospital are safe. Water births conducted in a home atmosphere are inherently not safe. The water and basin should be sterilized and should conform to OSHA standards. If an attendant and a support person are also in the water birth basin, more bacteria, possibly GBS, may be introduced and can contaminate the water. A second concern is the safety of an already unbalanced mom getting in and out of the tub and falling.

A water birth is supposed to relieve the pain of labor by immersing yourself in a warm, soothing bath. Studies, however, have shown that if pain relief is available, the mom will ask for it. If you believe that a water birth will help you through labor without analgesics, you have a 40 percent chance that it will. That's the percentage for the placebo effect, which is still good. Water births do not decrease the incidence of vaginal lacerations or tears.

CHAPTER 11

Cesarean Section

Q. *What is a cesarean section (C-section)?*

A. A C-section is a major surgical operation performed by your doctor to deliver your baby by an incision made through your abdomen into your uterus.

Q. *What are the indications for a C-section?*

A. The most common reasons for a C-section are the following:

- A previous cesarean section, if indicated or desired
- A cervix that fails to dilate completely
- A pelvis that is too small to allow the baby to descend through the birth canal
- Fetal distress due to an inadequate supply of oxygen to your baby
- An abnormal fetal position—breech (butt or feet first)
- Placenta previa
- Severe preeclampsia with an "unripe" cervix
- Diabetes with a large fetus (macrosomia)
- Uterine rupture
- Twins that are not both head down
- Triplets, quadruplets, and so on
- Prolapse of the umbilical cord through the dilated cervix

- Previous uterine surgery (for example, removal of a fibroid tumor)
- Pelvic tumor obstructing the birth canal
- Active genital herpes or a positive herpes culture at term
- Elective C-section

Q. *Who does the C-section?*

A. Your doctor performs the surgery, alone or with another doctor assisting, either his or her partner or an associate. Some obstetricians use a family doctor as an assistant.

Q. *What happens before I have the C-section?*

A. Your doctor will explain to you the reason for the C-section and the potential complications. You will then sign a consent form for the procedure. Your nurse will then prepare you for the surgery. A Foley catheter will be placed in your bladder to keep it drained; this is done to deflate it through the cut in the uterus and to prevent an injury to the bladder during the surgery. You will need an IV for hydration before the administration of the spinal or epidural anesthesia and for some medications, if needed, during surgery. The pubic hair on your abdomen will be shaved to clean the area where your doctor will make the incision. Blood will be taken for a CBC, blood type, and Rh titer to cross-match your blood in case a blood transfusion is necessary. A test will also be performed to see that your blood clots properly. If the C-section is not a life-threatening emergency for you or your fetus, the anesthesiologist will discuss the different types of pain relief that can be used during the operation. All this is done in the LDR.

You will then be transported to the operating room, usually located near the labor and delivery room, and moved onto the operating table. If a spinal or epidural anesthesia was selected, the anesthesiologist will place this now. If you already had an epidural for labor, more anesthetic will be given—a "C-section dose." General anesthesia for a C-section is rarely necessary, even in most emergency situations. You will lie on your back and your legs will be strapped down to prevent them from moving during the induction of sleep if general anesthesia is given or from falling off the table if a spinal or epidural was given. The anesthesiologist will monitor your blood pressure with a blood pressure cuff and your heart with electrocardiogram leads, which he or she will place on your chest. The oxygen level in your blood will be monitored with a pulse oximeter, a small device placed on your finger. A nurse will place a pad on your leg to ground you so that the doctor may use an instrument for cutting and cautery for hemostasis (to stop bleeding) during the procedure. Your abdomen will then be washed and sterile drapes will be placed over your body, except for the site of the incision.

Q. *Can I wear my contacts or glasses in the operating room?*

A. Yes.

Q. *Can I wear my earrings, necklace, bracelets, and watch in the operating room?*

A. Yes, as long as you are not undergoing general anesthesia. The hospital does not want to be responsible for your jewelry when you are not conscious.

Q. *Can my partner watch the C-section?*

A. Most doctors and hospitals allow the partner to be present during the cesarean section. He is usually asked to sit on a stool right by your head so that he may hold your hand and talk to you (if you are awake) during the surgery. A drape usually blocks his view of the surgery, but he can, if he chooses, stand up and watch any part of the C-section.

Q. *Can I watch the C-section?*

A. Some operating suites are equipped with mirrors, and these can be set up for you to view the surgery if you so desire.

Q. *Can we take pictures during the C-section?*

A. Absolutely.

Q. *Can we videotape the C-section?*

A. Most hospitals have a no-videotaping policy.

Q. *How is the C-section performed?*

A. First you will be prepped (cleaned with a type of soap) and draped. Your doctor will then test your skin for feeling. If you can feel a sharp or pinprick feeling, the anesthesiologist will administer more anesthetic if you have had an epidural. If you have had a spinal placed, it didn't work and a new one will have to be done. This is rare. If you are going to have a general anesthesia, this step is not necessary.

An incision is made with a scalpel (surgical knife) through the skin of the abdomen. Most commonly, the "bikini cut" is performed. The incision is made in a horizontal fashion from one side of your hip to the other. The length of the wound is from 4 to 6 inches long and is made about 1 inch above your pubic bone. The next layer entered is fat and looks yellow. The fascia, a white leathery covering, is cut next and then separated from the underlying abdominal muscles.

The muscles of the abdomen are separated, not cut, in your midline, and the peritoneum (the lining of the abdominal contents) is entered. Two metal instruments shaped like hoes are used to keep your belly open. The bladder is attached to the uterus. This attachment is cut and the bladder is pushed down away from the uterus. An incision is then made in this lower part of the uterus. Two types of uterine incisions can be made here, horizontal or vertical; the horizontal incision is more commonly made. The amniotic sac protrudes through this opening and is ruptured, with a gush of amniotic fluid pouring out. Your baby's head (or butt) is then delivered through this incision, the mouth is suctioned, and the cord is doubly clamped and cut (by your partner if desired). You will be shown your baby briefly, and then your baby will be placed in a warmer and dried and examined by a nurse and respiratory therapist. The placenta is delivered next. Blood is taken to test your baby. Pitocin is given through your IV to contract your uterus, and an antibiotic is given IV to prevent infection. The uterus is then brought out through the abdominal incision and placed on your belly. The uterus is wiped clean and then closed with suture. After noting that the incision is not bleeding, your doctor will look at your tubes and ovaries to make sure they are normal. The uterus will be replaced into your body and checked for bleeding and corrected with suture if necessary. The two sides of abdominal muscles will be sutured together and inspected for bleeding.

Next the fascia and fat layers will be closed. The skin incision can be closed with a suture just under the skin (my preference) or with staples. During the closure, you will be able to hold your baby.

Q. *How long does a C-section take?*

A. The average time is about 30 to 45 minutes. Your baby will be born within 5 minutes of the start of the C-section.

Q. *Who is in the delivery room during a C-section?*

A. There can be quite a few people: you, your mate, one other family member or friend (to take still photos), your doctor and his or her assistant, the anesthesiologist, your pediatrician, a scrub nurse to hand the instruments to the doctor, a labor nurse to get extra equipment (if needed), a nursery nurse, a respiratory therapist, and finally your new baby!

Q. *What are the potential complications of a C-section?*

A. Cesarean section has become one of the most common surgical procedures performed in this country. Over 25 percent of deliveries will be by C-section. Complications can and do occur, but they are extremely rare. In fact, a large recent study noted that all the types of complications from a C-section were only 17 per 1,000.

Any surgical procedure may cause an infection. Infections are more common in women who were in labor for hours with ruptured membranes before having a C-section, in diabetic women, and in women who are obese. The incidence of infections has decreased with the use of antibiotics given after the baby is born. Three types of infections may be seen: bladder infections, uterine infections, and wound infections.

Increased blood loss may occur after a C-section, especially if the mom was in labor for a long time and the uterus is too tired and doesn't want to contract (atony) or after delivery of multiple babies or huge babies. Placenta previa or accreta can cause a large blood loss. Although it has been stated that the blood transfusion rate can be as high as 6 percent, the rate in private hospitals is less than 1 percent.

Possible injury to other organs may occur in any surgical procedure; the most common is a bladder injury, which is rare. Adhesions or scar tissue may rarely form after any surgical procedure. In the case of a C-section, the scarring is usually between the uterus and bladder or between the uterus and the inside lining of the abdomen. Pain or discomfort from these adhesions is rare. Deep vein thrombosis (DVT), a blood clot in the leg, is rare, and women at greater risk for this will have prophylactic measures taken to prevent this complication.

Death of the mother is a very rare event, and there is usually some other complicating factor.

Q. *When will my skin incision be strong?*

A. At 2 weeks, the wound has about 10 percent of its strength, by 3 weeks 20 percent, and by 4 weeks 50 percent. You can take a shower and not worry the day after your C-section.

Q. *Is it normal to have numbness around the incision?*

A. Yes, some women will experience numbness, which may last for up to six months.

Q. *My incision was soft but now it feels hard. Is this normal?*

A. Yes, the skin and underlying tissues are undergoing a repair process that takes months. During the initial phases, the wound area may feel hard and swollen, which will disappear over the first few months.

Q. *Will I form a thick (hypertrophic) scar?*

A. Hypertrophic scars are thick scars that grow within the boundary of the incision. Most people confuse hypertrophic scars with keloids. These hypertrophic scars are more common in dark-skinned women or if you have a previous such scar on your body. They usually form in the first month after surgery and may subside over years. The thickness of the scars can be decreased with pressure and silicone sheeting.

Q. *Will I form a keloid scar?*

A. A significant factor for keloid formation, thick scars that extend beyond the incision, is a genetic predisposition. Asian women have a 50 percent chance; African-Americans have a 10 percent chance. The transverse abdominal skin incision has a lower probability of keloid formation than a vertical incision . Keloid formation usually develops several months after the surgery and rarely regresses. No good therapy is available.

Q. *When can I breast-feed my baby after a C-section?*

A. If an epidural or spinal block was used for anesthesia, you will be able to begin breast-feeding in the recovery room, after your vital signs have been taken. If you had general anesthesia, you will be groggy for about an hour after the surgery; but as soon as you are awake, you may start breast-feeding your baby.

Q. *What is a morphine epidural or spinal?*

A. A morphine epidural or spinal is a wonderful postoperative analgesic. After your baby delivers during the cesarean section, the anesthesiologist injects morphine through the catheter into the epidural space. The resultant effect is almost complete relief from pain for the ensuing 18- to 24-hour postoperative period. As the effect of the morphine wears off, the pain you will experience can usually be controlled by oral analgesics. If you have a spinal for anesthesia, the morphine is injected along with the anesthetic. The main advantage is the incredible lack of pain you will experience, which allows you to bond with and enjoy your baby immediately following your surgery.

Q. *What are the side effects of a morphine epidural or spinal?*

A. The side effects of the morphine epidural/spinal are minimal compared to the pain relief it affords you. You may experience nausea, which may be controlled by different medications. Pruritus, or itching, may be present, which also is usually easily treated. An oximeter must be worn for 12 hours and may go off frequently. This may be prevented by the use of nasal oxygen for the first 12 hours.

Q. *What happens to me after*
the C-section?

A. That night—as with a vaginal delivery—excitement and happiness may cause insomnia. Once in the recovery room, you will be reunited with your newborn. You will remain there for about an hour. Your vital signs will be checked constantly. Once you are stable and you stop shivering, you will be transferred to your postpartum room. Chew gum. This will stimulate your intestines to work and decrease the time it will take for you to pass gas and have a bowel movement. Your diet that day will begin with fluids and, if tolerated, solid food. Early feeding will also improve bowel function.

Start with small sips of fluids for about an hour. If you are not nauseous and, now hungry, you can start eating solid food. Begin eating as if you were at a party where hors d'oeuvres are being served. Have a small bite of your food every 10 to 15 minutes. This will ensure that you won't overdistend your stomach and vomit. Early feedings (along with early walking) will stimulate your intestines to work faster so you will have less gas and constipation. Your IV will remain in place for 18 to 24 hours. You will be allowed to shower as soon as the IV is removed; you may get your incision wet. The Foley catheter will be removed from your bladder on the morning of your 1st postoperative day. You will be asked to walk; early ambulation leads to early recovery! Your incisional pain and afterpains can be controlled with a combination of narcotic pills and ibuprofen. Your abdomen may become distended with intestinal gas on the 2nd or 3rd postoperative day, and you will look pregnant again. The best way to prevent this is to walk. I order nightly milk of magnesia until the new mom has a bowel movement. Most mothers have a bowel movement by the 4th postoperative day. Skin staples, if used, will be removed on the day you leave the hospital.

Q. *When can I leave the hospital?*

A. You can leave the hospital whenever you want. You may stay for 4 nights. Stay at least 2 nights.

Q. *Will there be much discomfort after my C-section if I have a general anesthetic?*

A. If you received a general anesthetic, you may experience some intense pain in the recovery room and for approximately the next 24 hours. You have undergone a major abdominal surgery, and this is painful. Of course, everyone has a different threshold for pain, so you will hear different impressions from your friends. The pain is most severe the day of surgery. The pain is more intense in women who were in labor and then required a cesarean section. Women who undergo planned repeat or planned primary cesarean sections do much better and feel better faster. Pain relief may be given in the form of intramuscular injections or via an intravenous line by a method called *patient-controlled anesthesia* (PCA) during the first 24 to 36 hours. Thereafter, oral medication for pain relief will usually suffice. By the time you leave the hospital, if it is on the 3rd or 4th postoperative day, you will be able to use a milder pain reliever.

Q. *What is PCA?*

A. PCA stands for patient-controlled anesthesia. A type of narcotic or nonnarcotic medicine is constantly infused at a low baseline rate. As needed, at certain prescribed intervals, you may give yourself a bolus (concentrated dose) of medication for the relief of pain. The advantages of this route of delivery are that you do not have to wait for a nurse to come in and give you an injection, you are not receiving intramuscular injections, you are receiving less of a dose of medication at a time, and therefore the side effects (nausea, dizziness, and somnolence) are minimized. The disadvantage is that the interval of time of pain relief is quite short, and if you sleep too long, you may wake up in intense pain and the bolus dose offered will not adequately relieve your pain.

Q. *I am scheduled for a repeat cesarean section. What should I do if I think that I am in labor?*

A. If you are experiencing uterine contractions every 8 to 10 minutes lasting 60 seconds and think you are in labor, so does your doctor; go to the hospital. If you think that you broke your bag of water, don't wait for contractions; go to the hospital. Don't eat or drink before you go; you will be having a repeat cesarean soon.

Q. *Is there a limit to the number of cesarean sections I can have?*

A. Yes. The major limitation is the number of children you want to have. There is really no increased risk of uterine rupture with subsequent pregnancies and cesarean sections. There is an increased risk of placenta previa with each successive C-section. The incidence may be as high as 3 percent after your fourth C-section. This means that 97 percent of the time, the placenta will not be a previa. Placenta accreta is also more common with each repeat C-section but still extremely rare. There may be a small to significant amount of scar tissue between your uterus and your abdominal wall. You will be unaware of these adhesions. The incision-to-delivery time will be slightly delayed.

Q. *I had a cesarean section with my first baby. Do I need to have another cesarean section, or can I try to deliver vaginally?*

A. The rule "once a cesarean, always a cesarean" does not now apply to everyone. If certain criteria are met, you may elect to have a trial of labor. The criteria are:

- The incision on the uterus was in the lower segment and made transversely.
- The reason for the previous cesarean section has not occurred in the present pregnancy (for example, placenta previa or breech presentation).
- The fetus weighs under 9 pounds.
- There is a clinically adequate pelvis—which means that the mom has had a previous successful vaginal delivery, because there is no other way to estimate whether the average woman will or will not delivery vaginally.
- The doctor must be readily available throughout the active stage of labor.
- All necessary personnel must be available for a possible C-section.

Q. *Are VBAC (vaginal birth after cesarean) deliveries common?*

A. No. The shift in recent times has been a decrease in the VBAC rate. The VBAC rate was about 9 percent in 2004.

Q. *If my first C-section was for CPD (cephalopelvic disproportion),*

*how good are my chances of delivering
vaginally in my current pregnancy?*

A. Your chances of having a normal delivery will be up to 66 percent.

Q. *If my C-section was for a breech,
what are my chances?*

A. Up to 90 percent of women will be able to deliver vaginally.

Q. *If my C-section was for fetal distress,
what are my chances?*

A. From 70 to 85 percent of women will have a normal delivery.

Q. *What are the dangers of a VBAC?*

A. The major risk is rupture of the uterus. It occurs about 1 percent of the time. It's not too common, but if it happens, the results may be catastrophic for both baby and mom. The baby could suffer from the long-lasting effects of oxygen deprivation, and the mom may require multiple blood transfusions. If the VBAC attempt is unsuccessful, there is an increased risk of infection in both baby and mom, low Apgar scores in your baby from decreased oxygen supply, and an increased blood loss due to uterine atony (the uterus is tired and doesn't contract fast).

Q. *What special procedures are done
during labor in a VBAC?*

A. Most hospitals have special policies for VBAC, such as:

- The laboring patient will have an IV.
- Internal monitors will be used during labor.
- The doctor must be in the hospital when the patient is in active labor.
- A consent form for C-section will be signed.
- Preoperative blood work will be drawn.
- Anesthesia coverage will be available for emergency C-section.

Q. *Do all doctors perform VBAC deliveries?*

A. No. There are many reasons why some doctors may not perform VBAC deliveries. Your doctor will not attempt a VBAC if your hospital does not have in-house 24-hour anesthesiology coverage or 24-hour in-house scrub tech coverage. Many doctors will not want to make the promise of a time commitment for a VBAC delivery. For example, if you had a previous breech delivery and this is your second delivery, your active phase of labor and second stage of pushing could last 6 or more hours. Honestly, not many physicians would want to be in the hospital during that time at night or on the weekends. There is no additional reimbursement for those hours spent.

ELECTIVE CESAREAN SECTION

Q. *I want to have a C-section and my only reason or indication is that I want one. Can I have a scheduled C-section?*

A. Yes. If you want an elective C-section, you may ask for one. Your doctor will go over the pros and cons with you. You will give proper informed consent for the procedure as well.

Q. *What are the benefits to an elective C-section for my newborn?*

A. There is about a 1 percent chance of oxygen deprivation to your baby during labor and delivery. The risk of a nonelective C-section for fetal distress accounts for about 10 percent of C-section deliveries. There is no risk of low-oxygen problems for the baby with a planned C-section. The perinatal mortality rates are nine times lower for elective C-section babies versus those delivered vaginally. The risk of shoulder dystocia and resultant Erb's palsy is virtually eliminated. The risk of bacterial and viral transmission is eliminated. There is absolutely no chance of a vaginal or perineal tear or laceration with resultant pelvic floor damage with an elective C-section. Elective C-sections are as safe to you as a vaginal delivery. The rates of DVT (deep vein thrombosis) and postpartum hemorrhage are the same for C-section and vaginal delivery.

Q. *What is the risk to my baby if I have a "maternal choice" C-section?*

A. Up to 2 percent of newborns may experience transient tachypnea (TTN), or rapid breathing. The baby may develop rapid breathing after delivery owing to less surfactant in the lungs of C-section babies at term. The rapid breathing resolves within 24 hours. Treatment is not necessary.

Q. *What are my benefits for choosing
an elective C-section?*

A. You do not have to have a vaginal delivery if you don't want
to. With C-section, there is no risk of vaginal trauma. The studies
about increased frequency of urinary incontinence, fecal incontinence, and change in sexual satisfaction after one or more vaginal
deliveries versus C-section are being compiled. Suffice it to say that
there is a difference, which will affect each woman differently.

CHAPTER 12

Postpartum

Q. *Should I stay in bed the whole day after having my baby?*

A. Yes, if you are exhausted from a long labor and delivery. Yes, if you had an extensive vaginal tear that is painful. Otherwise, no. Early walking will decrease your chances of bladder retention, constipation, gas pains, and blood clots in your legs.

Q. *Why do I still look pregnant after delivery?*

A. The day after delivery, your abdomen may still appear to be large, even though the top of your uterus is only up to your navel. Your abdomen may be distended with intestinal gas, which may happen with either a vaginal delivery or a cesarean section.

Q. *What can I do to reduce my bloating from gas?*

A. Bloating from intestinal gas is the norm. Chewing gum after delivery will stimulate your gut and hasten the return of normal bowel function. Do this after your baby is born and it will also serve another function—as a breath freshener. Over the next few postpartum days, walk around a few times per day, drink prune juice, eat foods high in roughage, and avoid foods that stimulate gas production (broccoli, cabbage, and beans). Medicines containing simethicone will also help relieve gas pains.

Q. *Can I use an abdominal binder?*

A. Sure, if the uterus flops forward and causes you discomfort, but a regular girdle will be just as helpful. Wearing a girdle will not help in the long run.

Q. *When can I start doing abdominal exercises?*

A. Now. You can start slowly by walking. Wait about 6 weeks after a C-section to do situps, stomach crunches, leg lifts, or pilates.

Q. *Is constipation a common problem postpartum?*

A. Constipation immediately postpartum is an all-too-frequent annoyance, which could turn into a really uncomfortable situation. If you were prone to constipation during pregnancy, it could be much worse in the immediate postpartum period. Laxatives may be used in this situation. I like milk of magnesia. It won't affect your baby if nursing. Difficulty with constipation may persist for the next nine months postpartum, but will not be to the same degree as experienced during your first week home. Constipation may be more common after a C-section if you remain in bed 24/7. Get up and move around. Sit in a chair. Constipation may be more common if you had a large vaginal tear, which is tender, or if you have tender hemorrhoids. The pain may make you afraid to have a bowel movement. Some women feel uncomfortable about having a bowel movement away from home and will have constipation in the hospital. Narcotics slow down bowel function and contribute to constipation.

Q. *How long will I have problems*
with my hemorrhoids?

A. Hemorrhoidal symptoms—itching, burning, bleeding, and
discomfort—will peak at about one month postpartum and may
continue at a moderate level of annoyance for the next two
months. Ask your nurse for Tucks, sprays, foams, and supposito-
ries. They are on your doctor's standard orders.

Q. *How should I take care of my*
episiotomy or vaginal /perineal tear?

A. Your nurses will show you how to clean your episiotomy site
after urinating. You will be supplied with a plastic squeeze bottle
with a curved nozzle, which is filled with soap and water and used
to douse this area. Remember to always wipe your perineum from
front to back and to use each piece of toilet paper only once.

Q. *What can I use to relieve the pain from*
the episiotomy or vaginal/perineal tear?

A. I like to have my patients wear an ice pack for at least 24 hours
after delivery if they have had an episiotomy. The cold decreases
the swelling that normally accompanies an injury (episiotomy in
this case) and also numbs this area, providing very good pain relief in most cases. At home you can use and reuse a bag of frozen
peas (or corn) that will nicely mold to your perineal area.

After the first day, a heat lamp or warm sitz (shallow-water)
baths for 20 minutes, three or more times a day, will help to minimize the discomfort. There are also anesthetic creams and foams
available to put on the episiotomy; your doctor will probably

order one of them as well as mild pain relievers. Ibuprofen around the clock to decrease inflammation and relieve pain is a great first option. Mild narcotic pills will be ordered as well.

Q. *Do I have to get the episiotomy*
stitches removed?

A. No. The sutures dissolve in 3 to 6 weeks. You may notice some pieces of suture in your lochia (discharge from your uterus), but don't worry, your vagina has already healed.

Q. *How long will I have discomfort*
from the episiotomy or vaginal tear?

A. It may bother you for a week or two or just a day or two. If the pain lasts longer or becomes worse, call your doctor. Some women have more pain from their hemorrhoids than from the episiotomy.

Q. *When can I have sexual intercourse*
after an episiotomy or vaginal/perineal tear?

A. Most of the time, your doctor will use sutures that dissolve in 3 weeks. Your episiotomy or tear will be sufficiently healed by then to resume sexual activity.

Q. *Can I walk up stairs if I had an*
episiotomy or vaginal/perineal tear?

A. Sure, but don't climb stairs two or three steps at a time. If the episiotomy site hurts when you climb stairs, limit the number of times you must use them during the day.

Q. *When is it safe to drive?*

A. Do not drive if you are still taking a narcotic pain reliever such as Darvocet (propoxyphen and acetaminophen) or Vicodin (hydrocodone and acetaminophen). You will be driving under the influence. That's a DUI.

Before driving, try these tests:

1. First, jump up and down. Too afraid? Then don't drive.
2. Second, if that was easy, then get in your car and pretend that you have to stop short. If your response time of your foot from the gas pedal to the brake pedal seems too slow because you are still tender, don't attempt to drive. Remember, most automobile accidents occur within 5 miles of your home.

Q. *Is it normal for my lower legs, ankles, and feet to swell postpartum?*

A. Yes. You may experience edema in your lower extremities starting a few days after birth that may last for up to 2 weeks postpartum.

Q. *What are "afterpains"?*

A. "Afterpains" are uterine contractions that may cause some discomfort after the delivery of your baby. This pain is more noticeable during nursing. Nursing stimulates your pituitary gland to release oxytocin, which, in addition to causing the muscle cells around your milk ducts to contract, will cause your uterus to contract. This will empty your uterus of any residual blood and tissue. The cramping pain is more common and more painful with subsequent pregnancies and may last for up to a week. Ibuprofen can be used initially, which is safe to use while breast-feeding. If you are very uncomfortable, ask your doctor for a mild narcotic-based pain reliever.

Q. *How long will I bleed postpartum?*

A. Whether or not you are breast-feeding, you may bleed for up to 8 weeks. The bleeding is heaviest the first few days after delivery and then may slow down only to start again with bleeding, spotting, or clotting. Or you may bleed for only a week.

Q. *When can I use tampons?*

A. Postpartum C-section moms can use tampons once they get home from the hospital. Postpartum vaginal delivery moms can use tampons whenever they can insert one without discomfort.

Q. *What is lochia?*

A. Lochia is the normal vaginal discharge you will experience during the first 6 to 8 weeks postpartum. The discharge is made up of blood and pieces of lining from your uterus along with your normal vaginal bacteria and discharge. The first few days after delivery, the lochia is red, owing to the blood from your uterus. After a few days or weeks, when the bleeding stops, the lochia is pale and yellow. After about 2 to 4 weeks, the lochia may turn white and have a characteristic and, to some, unpleasant odor. The lochia will disappear within 8 weeks.

Q. *I passed large clots. Is that abnormal?*

A. Passing clots may occur during the first few postpartum weeks and is normal. The slow discharge of blood from your uterus collects in your vagina and coagulates, forming a clot. Your vagina can expand to hold a large baby, so a clot the size of an egg is nothing to worry about. Typically, you will pass these clots when you increase your abdominal pressure, which will force the clot out of your vagina. This may occur when you cough, sneeze, get out of bed, or have a bowel movement.

Q. *What kind of bleeding is abnormal?*

A. A heavy flow of fresh, bright red blood is abnormal, and you should notify your doctor immediately. If the bleeding is so heavy and rapid that you are filling up a pad or tampon in an hour, call your doctor. This is a rare occurrence. If it does happen, however, it will appear about 2 to 4 weeks after delivery and is due to slow healing of the placental site or retained placental tissue. Treatment with Methergine and/or antibiotics will usually stop the bleeding, although a D&C is sometimes necessary.

Q. *Should I prepare my nipples*
for breast-feeding?

A. No special preparation is necessary to ready your nipples for breast-feeding. A study has shown that pregnant women who prepared only one nipple, by either rubbing, rolling, massaging with creams, or pulling, reported no difference in sensation between the prepared and unprepared sides.

Q. *How long will it take for my milk to come in?*

A. The appearance of breast milk may occur anytime after delivery for up to 10 days. The milk usually appears on the 3rd to 5th day after delivery. In the meantime, your baby will nurse on colostrum.

Q. *What is colostrum?*

A. Colostrum is a thick white or yellow liquid produced by your breasts by the 1st or 2nd postpartum day. Colostrum is made up of fat, protein, vitamins, and antibodies. These antibodies will protect your baby from bacterial and viral infections. Your breast will continue to secrete colostrum for up to 5 days.

Q. *What is breast fever?*

A. About 3 to 5 days after birth, both your breasts will become hard, engorged, and tender. You may feel warm and have a temperature of less than 100°F for less than a day. The fever will break with the first letdown of milk.

Q. *Can I breast-feed if I have inverted nipples?.*

A. Sure. If you have inverted nipples, you can use the Hoffman technique to evert them. Starting at about 34 weeks, place your index fingers at the edges of your areola and press it inward and away from your nipple. Move your fingers 90 degrees away and repeat. Do this twice a day.

Q. *Do I have to feed my newborn infant*
any other foods if I am breast-feeding?

A. Human milk is the most appropriate nutrient for your baby,
according to the American Academy of Pediatrics. The American
College of Obstetricians and Gynecologists believes that breast
milk alone will provide all the nourishment required for most babies during the first four to six months of life.

Q. *What are some other advantages of*
breast-feeding for me and my baby?

A. Breast-feeding is economical; you don't have to buy it. It is
easy to transport your baby's food around with you. It is convenient—there is always a supply, there is nothing to prepare, and it is
always at the correct temperature. Breast-feeding helps contract
your uterus and shrink it back down to its prepregnancy size faster.
Breast-feeding also works as a natural contraceptive agent to some
degree. Breast-feeding will burn calories, so with a well-balanced
diet, you will lose weight faster than with bottle-feeding. Breast-
feeding will protect you from some cancers. And with breast-feeding, you will bond in a special way with your baby.

Breast milk offers your baby immunological protection
against many types of diseases, allergies, and infections. Breast-fed
babies are ill less often and are hospitalized less for infection than
formula-fed babies. Breast-fed babies are not as likely to become
obese. These babies have less colic, gas, and constipation. The risk
of SIDS (sudden infant death syndrome) is lower in breast-fed infants. The protein and fat are more easily digested.

Q. *If I have small breasts, will I produce enough milk to properly nourish my baby?*

A. Yes. The size of your breasts does not matter. Breasts are mostly made up of fat—the larger the breasts, the more fat content. Breast milk does not come from breast fat. Breast milk is made from the breast glands, which make up only a small part of the breast. Breast glands enlarge during your pregnancy and after delivery, however.

Q. *How should the baby suck on my breasts?*

A. Start breast-feeding your baby as soon as he or she has warmed up after delivery. If this is your first baby, ask your nurse to show you how. Your baby should suck on as much of the areolar area as he or she can so that the milk is emptied from the ducts. The strength of the suction is not important; very little force is required to empty the breast reservoirs.

Q. *How can I prevent sore nipples?*

A. You can prevent soreness by having your baby suck on the areola and not just the nipple. Also, insert your finger into the corner of your baby's mouth to break the suction after feeding.

Q. *How often and how long should I breast-feed at each feeding?*

A. Most breast-fed babies should be nursed every 3 to 4 hours during the first month. Usually, he or she will let you know that it is time to eat. But if not, you should try to feed your baby at least six times a day. At the beginning, limit your feedings to 5 or 6 minutes on each breast, then gradually increase to 10 or 12 minutes per breast. The baby gets most of the breast milk during the first 6 to 7 minutes of the feeding. After a while, you may want to nurse for longer periods of time. Some mothers like to nurse, and some babies like to suckle. If you don't have the additional time, have your baby use a pacifier. You do not have to feed the baby any additional food or water; breast milk is enough.

Q. *How can I increase my supply of breast milk?*

A. First, if you think you do not have enough milk, call your pediatrician and discuss this. If your pediatrician agrees that you should increase your milk stores, then step up your feedings to every 2 hours during the day and at least every 3 hours at night. Also, try to get a little more rest and drink more fluids. After a few days, you will have more milk with each feeding. There is no specific food or beverage that will increase the quantity or quality of your breast milk.

Q. *Can I diet if I am breast-feeding?*

A. Yes, you can. Once your milk supply is in, you may start a weight loss diet. If your goal is losing 1 pound per week, you will continue to have an adequate milk supply and your baby will continue to grow. A diet of 1,800 calories a day will provide you with optimal milk production.

Q. *Can I work out while I am breast-feeding?*

A. Yes. Start slowly unless you had been exercising during your pregnancy. Aerobic exercise will not decrease your milk supply as long as you maintain a proper diet and keep well hydrated.

Q. *Should I avoid certain foods when I am breast-feeding?*

A. No, not in the beginning. There are really very few foods that will disturb your baby. After a few weeks, if you suspect that one particular food or spice is upsetting your baby, eliminate it from your diet.

Q. *Should I continue to take my prenatal vitamins while I am breast-feeding?*

A. If you are not eating a well-balanced diet, then vitamin supplementation is necessary. There is an increased need for folic acid, vitamin B_6, calcium, zinc, and magnesium. A true vegetarian diet excluding all animal products requires supplementation with vitamin B_{12}, zinc, and vitamin D.

Q. *How rapidly may I lose the rest of the weight I gained during my pregnancy if I am breast-feeding?*

A. If you are about average weight and lactating, a 2-pound-per-month weight loss will not affect your milk volume. If you are overweight, you may lose 4 pounds per month safely. Exercise is a wonderful way to complement your diet program.

Q. *Can I drink products containing caffeine when I am breast-feeding?*

A. You should drink a maximum of three cups of a caffeine-containing beverage. Any greater intake of caffeinated beverages may cause an irritable, awake infant (which can be very distressing, especially at 3 A.M.) and may decrease the infant's ability to absorb iron. Of course, if you think your child is jittery or restless with even a small amount of caffeine intake, stop drinking it.

Q. *Should I discontinue breast-feeding if I catch a cold or the flu?*

A. No, breast milk will not transmit these viruses to your baby. These infections are transmitted by water droplets from your nose or mouth. The baby will become sick, whether you breast-feed or bottle-feed, if you are not careful about preventing transmission of your germs.

Q. *If I am under stress or have a lot of anxiety, will my milk dry up?*

A. No, your emotional state will not interfere with your milk production. However, it may be harder for your milk to come down. If you are having this problem, sit or lie down for a few minutes before you breast-feed, and relax.

Q. *If I am having problems breast-feeding, whom can I call for help?*

A. Call your pediatrician first. If you need additional help, try La Leche League International. This organization has chapters all around the country. Their website is lalecheleague.org. You can also try the American Academy of Pediatrics at aap.org.

Q. *I am now 8 weeks postpartum and breast-feeding and my vagina is still tender when I have sexual intercourse. Is this normal?*

A. Yes, this is very common. This discomfort may be experienced by breast-feeding moms even if they had a C-section or did not have an episiotomy or vaginal tear. The tenderness is caused by a lack of estrogen in your body. This lack of estrogen is due to breast-feeding and the hormonal interplay necessary to produce lactation. The vaginal mucosa (skin) is dependent on estrogen for growth and will remain thin and tender for two to four months postpartum.

Q. *If I am breast-feeding, do I have to use contraception?*

A. Only if you don't want another child right away! Full breast-feeding will provide more than a 98 percent chance of protection from pregnancy during the first six months postpartum. The definition of full breast-feeding is that the infant's total suckling stimulus is directed to the mother's breast and is not diminished by the use of supplemental feeding or the use of a pacifier. Even with full breast-feeding, it is recommended that a contraceptive method be started by the end of the third postpartum month.

If you are breast-feeding and supplementing or allowing your infant to use a pacifier to satisfy suckling needs, a contraceptive method should begin no later than the end of the 3rd postpartum week if early resumption of intercourse is anticipated. If you are breast-feeding and menstruating, your risk of pregnancy without contraception may be as high as 36 percent at six months and 55 percent at twelve months postpartum. If no menstruation occurs, the pregnancy rates are as low as 3 percent at six months and 6 percent at twelve months.

It is also possible for you to ovulate before you experience your first menstrual period. This means that you could be pregnant for a time period before you realize that you began ovulating. If you are not planning to increase the size of your family right away, talk to your doctor about contraception before you leave the hospital.

Q. *What kind of contraception can I use when I am breast-feeding?*

A. You may use a barrier form of contraception, such as condoms, a diaphragm, the sponge, or an IUD or the minipill, Depo-Provera, or Norplant. These are all effective means of contraception that can be safely used while you are breast-feeding.

Q. *I am breast-feeding and I just found out that I am pregnant. Do I have to stop breast-feeding my baby?*

A. No. You may continue to breast-feed throughout your pregnancy, although about 50 percent of infants will wean themselves from the breast at some point during this pregnancy. There is a sharp reduction of breast milk during the second trimester, which may be the cause of this weaning. There is no increased incidence of miscarriages, preterm labor, stillbirths, or birth defects due to breast-feeding. The most common complaints are breast pain, fatigue, and irritability. If you do continue to breast-feed, you will need to increase your nutritional requirements appropriately to meet the caloric demands of both your new pregnancy and your milk production.

Q. *Can I breast-feed if I have had previous breast surgery?*

A. Most women can. Your plastic surgeon will have avoided cutting your milk ducts during breast implant or reduction surgery. Breast biopsies rarely cause a problem.

Q. *I want to breast-feed my baby, but I will have to go back to work in 6 weeks. What can I do?*

A. During your first 6 weeks postpartum, you may breast-feed your baby on demand or on a schedule. When you return to work, you can use a breast pump to save milk for your baby's daytime feedings. Breast milk is bacteriologically safe at room temperature for up to 8 hours. Breast milk can safely be stored in the refrigerator for up to 5 days unless it smells sour. It can also be stored in a self-defrosting freezer for six months and in a deep freeze for twelve months. Thawed breast milk should be used within 48 hours. There will be very little loss of nutrients and antibodies when milk is frozen and thawed.

Q. *What should I do for cracked nipples?*

A. To prevent cracked nipples, wash your breasts with water only. Soap can dry out the skin. Some mothers pat their breasts dry, express some milk, and let it air dry on the nipples. The fat content in the milk will keep the nipples soft. If your nipples are cracked, apply lanolin or some other commercial breast cream that does not have to be washed off before feedings. If you are allergic to wool, do not use lanolin; it is made from wool.

Q. *What are the signs of a breast infection?*

A. Breast infections or postpartum mastitis may occur anytime during the months that you breast-feed. You can develop a high fever (101ºF to 103ºF), and a portion of your breast will become hot, red, and tender.

Q. *What is the treatment for postpartum mastitis?*

A. This infection is easily treated with antibiotics. Only one duct is infected, so your baby will not become infected if you breast-feed.

Q. *I want to bottle-feed my baby. What can I do to stop my milk from coming in?*

A. Wear a snug-fitting, well-supporting bra (your pregnancy bra) day and night and avoid nipple stimulation. This will prevent lactation, but engorgement (swelling) of your breasts will occur, especially between the 3rd and 5th day after delivery. This engorgement may be very uncomfortable in up to 30 percent of mothers, but it may be controlled with the use of ice packs on your breasts and the use of a mild pain reliever. It takes about 2 weeks for the milk glands to dry up in a minority of moms. Keep a snug bra on until your breasts are not engorged. Do not try to express milk to relieve the tension. This may provide temporary relief, but it will stimulate your breast to produce milk.

Q. *I started breast-feeding, but now I want to stop. How can I dry up my breast milk?*

A. Wear a tight, supportive bra, and avoid nipple stimulation. The birth control pill may also be used to dry up your milk while providing an excellent method of contraception.

Q. *If I am bottle-feeding, when will I ovulate and have my first period?*

A. Ovulation rarely occurs before 6 weeks after delivery; however, it can occur as early as 3 weeks postpartum. Remember, you do not have to have a menstrual period before your first ovulation.

Q. *If I am bottle-feeding, when can I start taking a combination oral contraceptive pill?*

A. Non-breast-feeding women may start the combination birth control pill during the 3rd week postpartum. In fact, you should start any form of contraception during the 3rd week after delivery. You may also use the pill even if you had gestational diabetes during your pregnancy. Pregnancy-induced hypertension does not disqualify your use of the birth control pill either. If your blood pressure is back to normal by the 3rd week postpartum, you may begin the pill.

Q. *What is "rooming-in"?*

A. "Rooming-in" is offered by most hospitals. With this option, you have your baby with you 24 hours a day, and the baby does not go to the nursery. In some hospitals, your baby may be with you only when you are awake. The advantage of the modified plan is that it allows you to rest, take naps, and have visitors during your hospital stay. You will also be able to learn how to care for your baby with the help of the nurses.

Q. *Is it common not to sleep the first night after delivery?*

A. Yes. Even if you were in labor without sleep the previous night, you may not sleep much the night following delivery. You may be too exalted, too excited, and too happy to sleep. Don't worry, this is very normal. You will sleep well the next night. If it is difficult to sleep the next night—as sleeping in the hospital can be for any-one—ask for a sleeping pill; you will not become addicted, and it will not affect your baby.

Q. *What should I do in the hospital?*

A. Rest. Labor and delivery can be very strenuous, and you should rest up for your new routine at home. Just stay in bed or sit in a comfortable chair most of the day with your new baby and continue your bonding—holding, cuddling, and talking to him or her. Nurses will be in and out throughout the day to check your blood pressure, massage your fundus (top of your uterus), note the flow of your lochia, help you with breast-feeding, and answer any questions you may have. Some hospitals have parenting classes or videotapes that you can view. Visiting hours are usually from 12:30 P.M. to 8 P.M. Have fun showing off your baby. Limit the visitors the first day if you are too exhausted.

Q. *How long should I stay in the hospital?*

A. All insurance companies will allow a 2-night stay at your local "hotel hospital." Stay the 2 nights. You need the rest and may need the time to get acquainted with your new lifestyle.

Q. *Is it normal to experience hot flashes postpartum?*

A. Hot flashes are very common postpartum, especially if you are breast-feeding, although they may be common for the first month in non-breast-feeding mothers as well. Hot flashes are due to the hormonal changes that occur postpartum.

Q. *Is increased sweating common postpartum?*

A. Most new mothers will complain about increased sweating for the first three months postpartum.

Q. *What should I do on the first day I go home?*

A. Rest and enjoy your new baby. Many women tire easily from just packing to go home and unpacking when at home. This is normal. You may not feel up to visitors, so don't invite anyone. If a parent or other close relative wants to cook meals for you, great! Take advantage of everyone's goodwill and generosity. If you have other children at home, give them a good deal of attention, alone and with their new brother or sister, so they realize that you still love them as much as you did before the baby came home with you.

Q. *How soon after delivery can I*
have sexual intercourse?

A. If you had an episiotomy or vaginal tear, you should wait at least
3 weeks before attempting sexual intercourse. It takes 3 weeks for the
incision to heal properly. If you did not have an episiotomy, you may
resume sex after 3 weeks. The same goes for after a C-section. Intercourse, however, may be uncomfortable this early, because your vagina
has not returned to its former prepregnancy state. The skin in your
vagina may be very thin, especially if you are breast-feeding, and not
well lubricated. Be careful your first time, use a lubricant, and stop if
it is too uncomfortable. Many new parents are too tired to even think
about having sex for many weeks after bringing their new baby home.

Q. *How long will I have vaginal*
discomfort with intercourse?

A. If you are breast-feeding, this discomfort with intercourse usually will lessen by three months postpartum. However, about 20 percent of breast-feeding mothers will still have discomfort at one year.
Moms who do not breast-feed will not have the same degree of discomfort from lack of estrogen and will resume sex without discomfort as soon as 2 weeks after a C-section or vaginal delivery without a
tear or as soon as 3 to 6 weeks if a minor vaginal tear was sustained.

Q. *I had a vaginal delivery and now*
my vagina seems wider. Is this normal?

A. Vaginal delivery will cause stretching of the vagina and underlying muscles. The vaginal opening, mucosa, and muscles can become overstretched even without any tears. Multiple tears from

delivery can compound this relaxation. Your doctor is well aware of this and will repair you as best as possible. If after all your babies this relaxation in your vaginal outlet interferes with your sexual satisfaction, you may have it repaired.

Q. *How common is urinary incontinence after a vaginal delivery?*

A. Easily 25 percent of moms will experience loss of urine with coughing, laughing, sneezing, jogging, or lifting during the postpartum period.

Q. *What is anal incontinence?*

A. Anal incontinence is the involuntary loss of flatus (gas) or feces. Anal incontinence is common. Most women will have only mild symptoms, such as occasional loss of flatus. This will depend on your mode of delivery and the extent of your vaginal tears. For a C-section, it is rare. For a vaginal delivery:

- Without tears, up to 15 percent
- With second-degree tears, up to 25 percent
- With third- or fourth-degree tears, up to 50 percent

Q. *Are there exercises to tone my vaginal muscles?*

A. Kegel exercises will strengthen and tone the muscles of your pelvic floor. They may help tighten your vagina, which was stretched during birth. They will also tone your muscles to help control your urinary and anal incontinence.

Q. *When can I start doing Kegel exercises?*

A. As soon as you want to, as long as the exercises do not cause you any added discomfort.

Q. *How do I perform Kegel exercises?*

A. The best way to learn how to use the proper muscles for Kegel exercises is during urination. While urinating, squeeze your pelvic floor muscles to stop the flow of urine. Those are the muscles you will use. Now, anytime it's convenient during your day, squeeze and hold your pelvic floor muscles for at least 10 seconds. Repeat for fifteen sets, three times a day.

Q. *Is it normal to have a lack of desire for sex and have difficulty attaining an orgasm postpartum?*

A. Decreased desire for sex and difficulty reaching orgasm has been reported in at least 40 percent of postpartum women and may continue for the first six months postpartum. About 40 percent of these women will continue to have this problem for up to one year postpartum. This may occur in women who had either a vaginal or cesarean delivery. Discuss this with your partner.

Q. *When can I start exercising postpartum?*

A. You may start as soon as you feel up to it. If you were not exercising during your pregnancy, start very slowly, not more than 5 minutes per day, and gradually work your way up to a normal routine. Walking and swimming are excellent methods to slim down your waist. You may start swimming as soon as your bleeding has subsided.

Q. *When can I start abdominal toning exercises?*

A. Are you in the mood now? Go for it. Start all abdominal toning exercises slowly with low repetitions and ease of exercise. Leg slides are the easiest exercise to start with. Postpartum C-section moms can do these when their incisional pain has subsided.

Q. *When will I lose the weight I gained during my pregnancy?*

A. Following delivery, you will have lost the weight equal to the weight of your baby, placenta, and amniotic fluid. By the end of your 1st week postpartum, the excess water weight will also be shed. The extra weight of the uterus will be lost by one month postpartum. So by your first postpartum visit, without dieting, you will have lost about 80 percent of the weight you gained during your pregnancy (if you gained the recommended amount of weight). So if you gained about 27 pounds, you will have lost about 27 pounds, and if you gained about 47 pounds, you will have lost about 27 pounds.

Q. *I am about three months postpartum, and I think my hair is falling out. Can this really happen?*

A. Yes. It occurs in all postpartum women, to some degree or another. Pregnancy causes the continued growth of hair follicles, even those that should have stopped growing and fallen out. So postpar-

tum, with the effects of pregnancy now gone, many hair follicles
are shed. In some women, the hair loss can be marked. But rest as-
sured, new hair growth is occurring at the same time.

Q. *What are the postpartum blues?*

A. The postpartum blues, or the "baby blues," are a temporary
feeling of sadness, fatigue, irritability, sleeplessness, mood changes,
and hostility toward anyone and everyone, including your new
baby. Postpartum blues are different from postpartum depression,
which is a major psychotic disorder characterized by confusion,
disorientation, hallucinations, loss of all emotions, decreased activity, and a sense of helplessness and hopelessness.

Q. *How common are the postpartum blues?*

A. At least 80 percent of postpartum women experience them.
They may last only an hour or as long as a week. You may experience the blues anytime from the 1st day after delivery to three
months postpartum. Most commonly, this depressed feeling occurs between 3 and 5 days postpartum. In contrast, postpartum
psychosis is rare, occurring in 1 out of every 1,000 births.

Q. *What causes the postpartum blues?*

A. No individual factor can be pinned down as the cause. It is a
combination of factors:

- The rapid decrease in the levels of the hormones of
  pregnancy
- The unexpected feeling of fatigue after delivery

- The adjustment to a new sleep schedule, the episiotomy, afterpains, hemorrhoids, constipation, and breast tenderness
- The adjustment to being a mom and not just a daughter
- The adjustment to your postpartum body
- The sense of loss associated with not being pregnant, not being the center of attention, and not feeling as one with your baby
- Difficulty breast-feeding
- Guilt about not breast-feeding
- The apprehension about the responsibility of being a good mother and not just a milk dispenser

Q. *What are some common feelings and thoughts that new mothers may have?*

A. Common feelings and thoughts, prompted by postpartum blues but more likely to occur with PPD, include:

- Something is really wrong with me if I do not love my baby all of the time.
- If my baby is sick, everyone will think it is my fault.
- I should be able to make my baby happy all of the time. If I can't, then I am not a good mother.
- I should always put the needs of my baby first. The baby should always come first, even if I don't get proper rest, nutrition, and outside stimulation.
- I should know how to care for my baby instinctually.
- I should be happy about having the baby all the time. If I am not then I am bad.
- If people knew how upset I feel, they would think that I am a bad mother.

Q. *What should I do if I have the blues?*

A. As I mentioned before, the blues are temporary. If you have prepared yourself for them, you will recognize that this is what you are experiencing and you will be better able to cope with it. Discuss your feelings with your partner, mother, friends, and doctor. They will lend support and reassurance. If you are experiencing insomnia and have not slept for more than a day, ask for a sleeping pill and have your partner manage the night feedings. A good night's sleep will leave you refreshed and ready for motherhood. If the blues last for more than a week, a natural progesterone supplement may be administered for treatment.

Q. *What are the symptoms of postpartum depression (PPD)?*

A. Postpartum depression occurs in 10 percent of new moms. The symptoms can be mild to severe on any given day. PPD may begin up to a year after the birth. The most common symptoms are extreme fatigue, development of an eating disorder, insomnia, overwhelming sadness, and feelings of guilt. Panic attacks and feelings of anxiety are common. The mom will be overly concerned for her baby or can ignore the baby. Sometimes the mom will admit to wanting to harm her baby or herself.

Q. *What is the treatment for PPD?*

A. Call your doctor for referral to a psychologist or psychiatrist who specializes in treating this type of depression.

Q. *Who is at risk for postpartum depression?*

A. There are both obstetrical and psychological risk factors. The obstetrical risk factors are:

- Preeclampsia
- Polyhydramnios
- Difficult labor
- A multiple birth
- Preterm birth

The psychological risk factors are:

- History of psychiatric illness
- Family history of psychiatric illness, alcoholism, or drug addiction
- Current marital or family problems
- History of family conflicts
- Concurrent stressful life events
- A difficult psychological adaptation to the pregnancy

Q. *When does postpartum depression occur?*

A. You still have the blues after 2 weeks. Depression occurs most commonly during the 1st to 4th week postpartum, but it may occur anytime during the first three months postpartum. The sooner the psychosis begins, the more dramatic the symptoms are, but the recovery is usually quicker as well. Treatment is individualized.

Q. *If I had postpartum depression after my last pregnancy, what are my chances of having postpartum depression after this pregnancy?*

A. The chances of postpartum depression recurring in subsequent pregnancies is about 30 percent. A consultation with your psychiatrist in the third trimester to formulate a treatment plan is advisable.

Q. *What is postpartum psychosis (PPP)?*

A. PPP is rare. It will occur in only 1 in 1,000 postpartum women. The onset has no warning. It is sudden and severe, occurring in the 2nd or 3rd week postpartum. The mom will be delusional and suicidal and exhibit strange behavior. She may hallucinate and is definitely out of touch with reality. She will need immediate hospitalization at a psychiatric institute.

Q. *Are there any physical or psychological warning signs that I should notify my doctor about during the postpartum period?*

A. Yes. If you experience any of the following, call your doctor. Don't wait until your postpartum checkup:

- Vaginal bleeding that is a heavy flow of bright red blood, more than your normal menstrual period. You are bleeding enough to fill a tampon or a pad in an hour.
- Increasing tenderness, redness, and warmth in one section of your breast with fever of 100.4°F or above
- Abdominal pain with fever of 100.4°F or above and chills

- Increasing pain and tenderness at the episiotomy site
- Frequency and/or burning with urination
- Dizziness or fainting
- Severe, persistent headache
- Insomnia
- Severe depression

CHAPTER 13

Pregnancy in Women over Thirty-Five

Q. *If my partner is forty or older, does this increase my risk of having a child with Down syndrome or another congenital anomaly?*

A. Men who become fathers over the age of forty will have more offspring with certain autosomal dominant conditions, such as Marfan syndrome. Men over the age of forty-five are considered to be of advanced paternal age. There is an increased incidence of some X-linked disorders with dad's advanced age as well, which could potentially affect the next generation if a male. This is the "grandfather effect." The increase in risk, which could be twofold, will raise the risk from 1 in 10,000 to 1 in 5,000. The risk of having a child with Down syndrome is also increased after the age of forty-five.

Q. *Is my age a risk factor for having a miscarriage?*

A. Yes. The risk of having a miscarriage is about 15 percent before the age of thirty-five. Women aged thirty-five to forty-five have up to a 35 percent chance of miscarriage. If you are forty-five or older, your chance of miscarriage may be as high as 50 percent.

Q. *Do women over the age of thirty-five
have a higher incidence of preterm labor?*

A. Yes.

Q. *Do women over the age of thirty-five
have an increased incidence
of postdate pregnancies?*

A. No.

Q. *Do women over the age of thirty-five
have a higher incidence of
FGR during pregnancy?*

A. No.

Q. *Do women over the age of thirty-five
have a higher incidence of stillborns?*

A. Not if there is no superimposed medical problem.

Q. *Will my labor be longer if I am
thirty-five or older?*

A. No. The length of labor does not seem to be affected by the age of the mother.

Q. *Will I have more complications during
labor if I am thirty-five or older?*

A. If you are in good health, the course of labor and delivery should be no different from that experienced by your younger friends. However, if you are not as physically fit as your younger counterparts or if you do have medical problems, your chance of requiring a cesarean section for delivery is higher.

Q. *Do women over the age of thirty-five*
  have a higher incidence of large babies?

A. Yes. Large babies are twice as common in your age-group. The incidence of babies weighing over 9 pounds is about 7 percent.

Q. *Do women over the age of thirty-five*
  have a higher incidence of cesarean sections?

A. Yes, it seems that this does occur. In fact, in one recent report, the C-section rate was two times greater in women age thirty-five or more compared to women between the ages of twenty and twenty-nine. This increased rate of cesarean sections for first-time older moms may be due to increased concern over the outcome of the pregnancy by both the doctor and the mom. Moms over forty also have an increased risk of C-section due to arrest of dilation. This is due to aging of the muscle of the uterus

Q. *What medical problems are more*
  frequent in women over the age of thirty-five?

A. Hypertension, diabetes, heart disease, obesity, and uterine fibroids are all more common in women with advancing age. If you have one of these disorders, consult your doctor.

Q. *Is preeclampsia more common in women over thirty-five?*

A. Yes. PIH is 1½ times as common.

Q. *Is the risk of having a baby with spina bifida increased if I am thirty-five or older?*

A. No. There does not seem to be an age-related risk.

Q. *Are multiple births more common in women over the age of thirty-five?*

A. Yes. In fact, over 6 percent of pregnancies are twins or more in women over thirty-five.

Q. *What is Down syndrome?*

A. Down syndrome is a chromosomal disorder. Normally, each cell has twenty-three pairs of chromosomes. In Down syndrome, there is an extra chromosome with the twenty-first pair. This extra chromosome may cause a variety of abnormalities in the child, such as characteristic facial features, mental retardation (mild to moderate), and high incidence of heart abnormalities.

Q. *What is the risk of having a baby with Down syndrome if I am thirty-five or older?*

A. The risk of having a baby with Down syndrome at age thirty-five is 1 in 250. The risk of having a baby with any chromosomal abnormality (extra chromosomes besides on chromosome 21, deleted chromosomes, and so on) is 1 in 132. The risk of having a Down syndrome baby increases with age: about 1 in 70 at age forty and 1 in 20 at age forty-five.

Q. *How can Down syndrome be detected during pregnancy?*

A. As discussed previously in Chapter 7, "Special Tests," an increased risk for Down syndrome can be assessed by a series of non-invasive tests: the first-trimester screening of nuchal translucency plus biochemical marker blood tests performed at 11 to 14 weeks along with the AFP quad test drawn at 15 to 17 weeks and a second-trimester level II ultrasound at 18 weeks. The diagnosis of Down syndrome can be detected by chorionic villus sampling at 10 to 11 weeks or by amniocentesis at 15 to 18 weeks.

Q. *Are there many women pregnant over the age of thirty-five?*

A. Yes, and the numbers are rising. Currently, 1 in 5 women are over the age of thirty-five when they have their first child. There are approximately 4 million pregnancies every year. Moms over thirty-five account for 13.5 percent of births per year—that's over half a million babies a year!

Appendix

Support Groups

American Cleft Palate Educational Foundation
1504 E. Franklin Street, Ste. 102
Chapel Hill, NC 27514
1-800-242-5338
Web site: cleftline.org

American College of Obstetricians and Gynecologists
409 12th Street, SW
PO Box 96920
Washington, DC 20090-6920
1-202-638-5577
Web site: acog.org

American Society of Human Genetics
9650 Rockville Pike
Bethesda, MD 20814
1-301-634-7300
Web site:
http://genetics.faseb.org
/genetics/ashg/ashgmenu.htm

Association for Retarded Citizens
1010 Wayne Avenue, Ste. 650
Silver Spring, MD 20910
1-301-565-3842
Web site: thearc.org

Cystic Fibrosis Foundation
6931 Arlington Road
Bethesda, MD 20814
1-800-344-4823
Web site: cff.org

Fetal Alcohol Syndrome
NCBDDD, CDC
Mail-Stop E-86
1600 Clifton Road
Atlanta, GA 30333
1-800-232-4636
Web site:
cdc.gov/ncbddd/fas/default.htm

U.S. Environmental Protection Agency Fish Advisories
Jeffrey Bigler
1200 Pennsylvania Avenue, NW
4305T)
Washington, DC 20460
Web site: epa.gov/ost/fish

Fragile X Foundation
PO Box 190488
San Francisco, CA 94119
1-800-688-8765
Web site: fraxa.org

Little People of America
5289 NE Elam Young Parkway,
Ste. F-100
Hillsboro, OR 97124
1-888-572-2001
Web site: lpaonline.org

March of Dimes Genetic Counseling and Birth Defects Foundation
1275 Mamaroneck Avenue
White Plains, NY 10605
1-914-428-7100
Web site: marchofdimes.com

Muscular Dystrophy Association
National Headquarters
3300 E. Sunrise Drive
Tucson, AZ 85718
1-800-344-4863
Web site: mdausa.org

National Down Syndrome
Congress
1370 Center Drive, Ste. 102
Atlanta, GA 30338
1-800-232-6372
Web site: ndsccenter.org

National Huntington's Disease
Association
505 Eighth Avenue, Ste. 902
New York, NY 10018
1-800-345-4372
Web site: hdsa.org

National Marfan Foundation
22 Manhasset Avenue
Port Washington, NY 11050
1-800-862-7326
Web site: marfan.org

National Neurofibromatosis
Foundation
95 Pine Street, 16th Floor
New York, N. 10005
1-800-323-7938
Web site: ctf.org

National Organization of
Rare Disorders
55 Kenosia Avenue
PO Box 1968
Danbury, CT 06813-1968
1-203-744-0100
Web site: rarediseases.org

National Tay-Sachs &
Allied Diseases Association
2001 Beacon Street, Ste. 204
Brighton, MA 02135
1-800-906-8723
Web site: ntsad.org

National Tuberous Sclerosis
Association
8000 Corporate Drive, Ste. 120
Landover, MD 20785
1-800-225-6872
Web site: ntsa.org

Organization of Teratology
Information Specialists
UCSD Medical Center,
Department of Pediatrics
200 W. Arbor Drive,
Mail Stop 8446
San Diego, CA 92103-8446
1-800-532-3749
Web site: otispregnancy.org

Sickle Cell Anemia Foundation
6133 Bristol Parkway, Ste. 240
Culver City, CA 90230
1-877-288-2873
Web site: scdfc.org

Spina Bifida Association of
America
4590 MacArthur Boulevard
NW, Ste. 250
Washington, DC 20007-4226
1-800-621-3141
Web site: sbaa.org

Index